Incorporating
HERBAL
MEDICINE
into
Clinical Practice

D1563806

Incorporating
HERBAL
MEDICINE
into
Clinical Practice

ANGELLA BASCOM

MSN, ARNP
Family Nurse Practitioner
Clinical Herbalist
Therapeutic Touch Practitioner
Certified Clinical Hypnotherapist
Ashland, New Hampshire

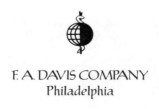

F. A. DAVIS COMPANY
Philadelphia

F. A. Davis Company
1915 Arch Street
Philadelphia, PA 19103

Printed in Canada

Last digit indicates print number: 10 9 8 7 6 5 4 3 2 1

Acquisitions Editor: Joanne Patzek DaCunha, RN, MSN
Developmental Editor: Catherine E. Harold
Production Editor: Jessica Howie Martin
Cover Designer: Louis J. Forgione

As new scientific information becomes available through basic and clinical research, recommended treatments and drug therapies undergo changes. The author and publisher have done everything possible to make this book accurate, up to date, and in accord with accepted standards at the time of publication. The author, editors, and publisher are not responsible for errors or omissions or for consequences from application of the book, and make no warranty, expressed or implied, in regard to the contents of the book. Any practice described in this book should be applied by the reader in accordance with professional standards of care used in regard to the unique circumstances that may apply in each situation. The reader is advised always to check product information (package inserts) for changes and new information regarding dose and contraindications before administering any drug. Caution is especially urged when using new or infrequently ordered drugs.

Library of Congress Cataloging in Publication Data

Bascom, Angella, 1956–
    Incorporating herbal medicine into clinical practice / by Angella Bascom.
        p. ; cm.
    Includes bibliographical references and index.
    ISBN 0-8036-0936-1 (pbk.)
        1. Herbs—Therapeutic use—Handbooks, manuals, etc. I. Title.
    [DNLM: 1. Plants, Medicinal—   therapeutic use—Handbooks. 2. Clinical Medicine—Handbooks.
QV 735 B298i 2002]
RM666.H33 B37 2002
615'.321—dc21

2001058272

With Thanks

This book was really written by my family—Jim, Zach, A. J., and Mark. All of them helped me by fixing the computer, doing laundry, preparing meals, motivating me, inspiring me, and giving much-needed emotional support. Thank you to Rosemary Gladstar, Mark Blumenthal, Dr. Andrew Weil, Robert McCaleb, and many others for helping me with my herbal education. I would also like to thank Dr. Rosita Arvigo of Belize for her passion for natural healing and her wonderful gift of helping other cultures save herbal knowledge and plants. Thank you to Steven Ottariano, pharmacist, herbalist, and friend; to my brother, John Thompson, the intuitive environmentalist and natural resources specialist; and to Mike Andruczyk, a wonderful botanist and friend. Special thanks for his help with taking many of the herb photographs. Finally, many thanks to all the scientists and herbalists who are coming together to heal the environment outside and inside all of us.

Author's Note

My interest in herbal medicine began about 15 years ago when my son developed a chronic skin rash. I tried over-the-counter ointments and received a much stronger ointment from our pediatrician, but neither of these treatments helped. It was then that I met an Ayurvedic practitioner, who gave me a homemade herbal ointment that cleared the rash in a day. That winter I had a cold and for the symptoms was given herbal teas, which helped my spirits along with my symptoms. Since then I have attended workshops, courses given by well-known herbalists, and presentations by leading health-care professionals to learn the scientific aspects of herb use. Living close to Shaker Village in New Hampshire, I am constantly reminded of the value of the historical use of herbs, and I have fond memories of my parents' use of folklore remedies for my healing.

I decided to write this book in response to nurse practitioners and nurses who have asked me for easy-to-read information on all aspects of herbal medicines. The book started as my Masters project when I was a student nurse practitioner. For that project, I focused on folk medicine in the United States and researched and devised a materia medica for 11 popular herbs. In this book, I have expanded my focus and added information about another 39 herbs. Although the book is intended for health care practitioners, I have also provided ample patient information that you may wish to copy and disseminate to patients as appropriate. Patients who have a strong interest in herbal medicine may prefer to purchase a copy of the book to gain access to the full range of information I have provided for each herb.

I hope you will use this book as an easy way to introduce yourself to the wonderful healing world of herbs. My intention is to give you a very brief overview of common herbal medicines from their historical uses to the results of scientific studies about them. I have included a large number of detailed and exhaustive articles and reference books on botany, pharmacology, and studies of herbs in the reference section at the end of this book.

Keep in mind that we are gaining knowledge about herbs daily, particularly regarding herb-drug interactions. Stress to your patients that the information sheets included in this book are not exhaustive and may not contain the very latest information. Naturally, if you learn of an herb-drug interaction not included on these patient information sheets, you'll want to write it down for your patients and yourself. Some herbs, especially when used with prescription medications, can have serious adverse effects.

Like a growing number of health care practitioners, I find myself in the interesting position of trying to merge herbal medicines with a modern health-care environment that relies on science, research, and technology. Although I do not believe that herbal medicines can or should supersede modern medicine, I do believe that herbal medicines may be able to replace many over-the-counter medications for patients who are not also taking daily prescription medications. As a health-care practitioner and practicing herbalist, I try to find a balance in integrating herbal medicines that have been used for centuries into the 21st century of medicine, nursing, and science. I commonly recommend herbal medicines, usually along with lifestyle changes. If herbal medicines do not work initially, I then refer the patient to another herbalist or prescribe a conventional medicine.

As a health-care professional, you will find many aspects of herbs to get excited about. Start your journey with five nontoxic herbs; get to know them by growing them; create an herbal salve; or investigate the growing scientific knowledge about a popular herb such as St. John's wort. Find out what your patients think of herbal medicines and what cultural traditions they practice in their homes. You'll be amazed at the important role herbs play in many cultures. Good luck in your herbal adventures.

Angella Bascom

Reviewers

JANET AUER, RN, MSN, FNP-CS
Assistant Professor
University of May
Bismarck, North Dakota

CYNTHIA L. BLEVINS, RN, MED, MSN, CRNP
Adult Nurse Practitioner
Chester County Cardiology Associates
West Chester, Pennsylvania

PATRICIA G. CHICHON, RN, MSN, APN-C
Nurse Practitioner, Homeopath, Herbalist
The Chrysalis Center
Lambertville, New Jersey

MAUREEN L. DEVER-BUMBA, RN, MSN
Assistant Professor, Coordinator of NP Programs
Medical College of Georgia
Augusta, Georgia

R. ERIC DOERFLER, MSN, NP
President, Nightingale Health Centers, Inc.
New Cumberland, Pennsylvania

BERNADETTE M. DRAGISH, RN, MSN, CFNP, PHD(c)
Associate Professor
Bluefield State College
Bluefield, West Virginia

DEBORAH GUTSHALL, RN, MSN, CRNP
OB/Gyn Nurse Practitioner, Pinnacle Health
Clinical Nursing Faculty, Harrisburg Area Community College
Harrisburg, Pennsylvania

JACQUELYN K. HOWELL, RN, PHD
Associate Professor in Nursing
Augustana College
Sioux Falls, South Dakota

MARY D. KNUDTSON, RN, MSN, FNP, PNP
Director, FNP Program
University of California, Irvine
Irvine, California

STEVEN G. OTTARIANO, RPH
Clinical Staff Pharmacist
Veterans Administration Medical Center
Manchester, New Hampshire

JANIS E. TOWN, MSN, FNP, CS
Family Nurse Practitioner
Cape May, New Jersey

Contents

CONTENTS

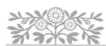

PART THREE

APPENDICES, REFERENCES, AND RESOURCES 296

INDEX 328

part 1

OVERVIEW

INTRODUCTION

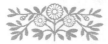

Herbal medicine has been used worldwide throughout history. In 1985 the World Health Organization (WHO) estimated that perhaps 80 percent of the world's people relied on herbs for their primary health-care needs (Akerele, 1992). India's Ayurvedic medicine and traditional Chinese medicine both include the use of herbal remedies, as do European and Japanese medicine. The German Federal Health Agency has researched more than 300 herbs and found them to have favorable benefit:risk ratios.

Colonists brought culinary herbs to America so that they could create kitchen gardens outside their homes. They also learned the value of many herbal medicines from Native Americans. Consequently, our ancestors were able to pass down valuable information for self-healing and comfort based on growing, preparing, and treating family members with herbs.

By the late 1990s, herbal medicines had grown to an estimated $5.1 billion industry in the United States (Eisenberg et al., 1998). This growth in herbal medicine comes from our own folk medicine practices, which have survived over the decades, and also from the health-care practices of many cultures now present in the U. S.

Another reason for this increased interest in herbal medicine is the rising cost of conventional (allopathic) medicines. Consider, for instance, the treatment of benign prostatic hyperplasia. It can cost $5000 (for surgery and its substantial risks); $2.17 per day (for Proscar, which carries a risk of impotence and is dangerous for patients with liver disease); or $0.86 per day for saw palmetto, which has no known side effects (McCaleb, 1996). To be cost effective, health care must also focus on disease prevention and health promotion. In other countries, echinacea and ginseng have been used safely to promote health by fighting stress and boosting the immune system.

This is not to say that all herbal products are safer than conventional drugs. Some herbs are toxic and others have increased side effects as their dosages are increased. Also, when patients combine herbal products with conventional medicines, herb-drug interactions can occur. Therefore safety and quality control are a concern for both patients and health-care professionals. In 1993 the National Institutes of Health (NIH) established an Office of Alternative Medicine (OAM) to evaluate and establish grants for research into alternative medicine, including herbal medicine (Weisman, 1994). In 1999 the NIH expanded the OAM into what it is now: the National Center for Complementary and Alternative Medicine. The mission of this agency is to stimulate,

3

develop, and support research on complementary and alternative medicine for the benefit of the public. Even within health-care professions, complementary and alternative medicine is creating increased interest and information. For example, the entire November 11, 1998 issue of the *Journal of the American Medical Association* was devoted to alternative medicine.

With the evolution of a more global society and increased access to information from other countries and cultures, we find ourselves in the midst of an incredible time of change in the practice of herbal medicine. This book will serve as an introduction to this ancient but rapidly changing field.

chapter one

HERBAL MEDICINES: AN HISTORICAL OVERVIEW

The World Health Organization (WHO) defines herbal medicines as "Finished, labeled medicinal products that contain as active ingredients aerial (above ground) or underground parts of plants, or other plant material, or combination thereof, whether in crude state or as plant preparations" (WHO, 1991). McCaleb and collaborators (2000) define herbs as "Plants or plant parts that are used in fresh, dried, or extracted form for promoting, maintaining, or restoring health." Bown (1995) writes, "Botanists describe an herb as a small, seed-bearing plant with fleshy, rather than woody, parts" and adds that "herbs are valued for their flavor, fragrance, medicinal and healthful qualities, economic and industrial uses, pesticidal properties, and dyes."

Although these are modern definitions of herbal medicines, healers and naturalists around the world have been using herbs in keeping with these definitions for centuries. Indeed, they have long recognized in herbs a vibrant essence and potential for healing. From the time of Paracelsus to today's modern world, doctors and scientists have explored the mysteries of natural herbal medicine.

EVOLVING VIEWS OF HERBAL MEDICINE

One physician who came to prominence in London in the 1930s was Edward Bach. Adhering to the doctrine of Paracelsus, who encouraged physicians to search within themselves for spiritual insights about the dynamics of herbs, Bach experimented with plants and found that those with high vibrations (energy frequencies) could raise lowered human vibrations and thus improve health. He was convinced that "herbal remedies have the power to elevate our vibrations, and thus draw down spiritual power, which cleanses mind and body, and heals." From Bach's point of view, herbal remedies share the same power as any spiritually uplifting medium, be it music, art, or scent. Bach's research contradicted contemporary Western medicine. Instead of trying to kill or destroy a disease, Bach flooded the body with beautiful vibrations from wild flowers and herbs, saying that in their presence "disease would melt away as snow in the sunshine" (Tompkins & Bird, 1973, p. 307).

In Native American tradition, it is not simply the energy force that a plant gives out that is beneficial, but the sacred relationship between the plant and the person

5

seeking to use the plant that provides the healing power. Chippewa medicine men, for example, made an offering of their cherished tobacco when gathering herbs and plants for medicinal purposes. By giving something precious, the Chippewa entered into a reciprocal relationship with the plant whose healing power they wished to extract (Griggs, 1981). The Native Americans' pantheistic view of nature holds that mind, body, and spirit are inseparable, and that all animals, plants, and living creatures are infused with spiritual life (Griggs, 1981).

Paracelsus, Native Americans, and many cultures today have shared the view of the Doctrine of Signatures, which means that a plant offers clues to its medicinal qualities. The clue could be the color or the shape of the plant. For example, the red hibiscus flower (red representing blood according to the Doctrine of Signatures) has been used in other cultures to treat postpartum hemorrhage. Another example is ginseng root, which resembles the human shape and is believed to benefit overall health.

Herbal traditions of colonists in early America initially involved culinary herbs, which they brought with them and planted in their kitchen gardens. But the colonists were intrigued by the Native Americans and their freedom from disease. Among the many cultural interchanges between colonists and Native Americans was knowledge of the key medicinal uses of indigenous plants (plants growing naturally in the environment). Indeed, some herbs (sassafras, tobacco, and ginseng) used medicinally by Native Americans became part of the white man's economy. By 1820, when the first *U. S. Pharmacopeia* was published, 130 of the 296 substances listed were remedies with Native American origins (Vogel, 1970).

Many physicians of that time observed Native American practices and incorporated herbal medicines into their own practices. As in Western medicine, Native Americans used particular herbal remedies to address particular disease processes: poke root was used as a poultice for skin cancer; snakeroot was used for snakebite and pulmonary ailments; and lobelia was used for syphilis (Vogel, 1970). The Cherokees discovered that pinkroot was an excellent cure for worms. "A century later, powdered pinkroot was a standard treatment for children with worms and was found in virtually every druggist's shop" (Griggs, 1981, p. 133). Natural elements that Native Americans used to suppress ovulation and control the menstrual cycle eventually contributed to the development of oral contraceptives centuries later. Another example of their advanced knowledge was their use of molds and fungi. Although they were perhaps unaware of how and why molds functioned in health care, they were doubtless employing the basic principles of modern-day antibiotics (Vogel, 1970, pp. 4–5).

Women, who were the predominant healers and herbalists before the turn of the 20th century, were the first to incorporate Native American remedies into their own repertoires of herbal solutions to sicknesses and afflictions. Before the 1860s, most families were treated by women who collected their home remedies from nearby woods and streams or grew them specially in their gardens (Caplan, 1989). One of these women, Martha Ballard, is described in detail in an historical account by Ulrich (1991, p. 53). Martha's diary, written in the late 1700s, offers a glimpse of what healers like herself believed medicine to be. She writes, "Nature offers solutions to its own problems. Remedies for illness can be found in the earth, in the animal world, and in the human body itself."

In the 1700s and 1800s, medical care was unavailable to many families in rural areas, and this is still the case today. Alternative health-care movements arose at that time as a result of this lack of access to medical care. One of these, the Thomsonian movement, was led by New Hampshire native Samuel Thomson in the early 1800s. Thomson patented a system of herbal medicine that, in 1839, claimed more than 3 million faithful followers. Other movements in health care arose that rivaled the influence of physicians (known at that time as Regulars).

Homeopathy and Eclecticism were founded at this time as well. Homeopathy differed from Western medicine in that it used tiny amounts of plants, minerals, or animal substances to treat conditions by promoting inner healing without harmful side effects. Many patients were drawn to the gentleness of these remedies. Eclectics (physicians who used herbs and other natural therapies) wild-crafted (picked plants in their natural surroundings) or ordered their herbs from the Shakers in New Hampshire. Many Eclectics created their own plant medicines and tried to educate the Regulars about herbal medicine.

THE DECLINE OF HERBS AS MEDICINES

In the 1820s, an Eclectic physician named John King discovered the full spectrum of a plant's function through what he called concentrated principles. This idea excited pharmaceutical company founders because they recognized the potential of breaking plants down, isolating their active components, and "producing even more powerful drugs in standard form" (Griggs, 1981, p. 233). Although it opened the door to the standardized medicines we use today, this exciting discovery also sparked a decline in the use of plants for medicinal purposes.

Another factor leading to the decline of herbal medicine in the U. S. was the idea that medicine was not valid if it did not have a scientific basis. Changing financial backing helped to further this idea. Alexander Flexner, an educator with a bachelor's degree from Johns Hopkins and the brother of the president of the Rockefeller Institute for Medical Research, was hired by the Carnegie Foundation to evaluate medical schools and their curricula and to provide appropriate medical schools with funds. Concurrently, the Rockefeller General Education Board (and other foundations) awarded $91 million to certain medical schools—primarily those that were founded for scientific research rather than medical practice (Starr, 1982). Many other types of medical schools and Eclectic schools were forced to close from lack of funds. The curriculum in existing medical schools was changed to eliminate botany and pharmacognosy and to add pharmacology, which focused on diseases and cures rather than on health and prevention. Nutrition was limited to its relationship to pharmacology.

Over time, the use medicinal plants fell out of vogue and was replaced by surgery, anesthesia, and transfusion and injection techniques. Pharmaceutical companies exploded with new discoveries of both drugs (penicillin, sulfonamides, and so forth) and vitamins. They also discovered that chemical monosubstances were profitable, convenient, and could be protected by patent, unlike herbal medicines, which were available to anyone, needed to be picked at the right time, and needed to be dried and stored properly to preserve the active chemical constituents of the plant.

Still, plants continued to be investigated and considered noteworthy by those who witnessed their healing properties. One plant that was noted to have amazing properties was garlic. Dr. W. Minuchin, a physician who was interested in the effects of garlic, performed clinical trials and found that garlic was useful in treating tuberculosis, lupus, diphtheria, and infections. However, because garlic was not a chemical monosubstance and could not be patented or made profitable, it was not considered worth pursuing as a treatment (Griggs, 1981).

Another reason for the increased emphasis on chemical monosubstances was the need to recover the cost of developing a new chemical compound for a drug. This cost for a single chemical compound, according to a 1990 report noted in Tyler (1993, p. 11), was "$231 million over a period of 12 years." Today a new prescription medication in the United States costs an average of $350 million in research expenses (Bauer, 2000). Many of the new conventional drugs can recover these expenses over a patent life of 11 years, unlike plant products, which are difficult to harvest, standardize, and store properly to maintain the active compounds.

A MODERN RESURGENCE

Despite these obstacles, herbal medicines have made a dramatic comeback in popularity over the last few years. Some of the reasons for this resurgence are discussed in the introduction to this book. In 1996, Brevoort reported that the top 10 herbs sold in selected health food stores in the U.S. were echinacea, garlic, goldenseal, ginseng, ginkgo biloba, saw palmetto, aloe, ma huang, Siberian ginseng, and cranberry. These statistics were based on a 1995 survey of 163 stores done by Richman and Witkowski for *Whole Foods* magazine. In 1998 and 1999, Blumenthal (2000, p. 47) reported a similar "top 10" that included ginkgo biloba, St. John's wort, ginseng, garlic, echinacea, saw palmetto, soy, horse chestnut, and cranberry.

Throughout the 1990s, herbal medicine sales in the U.S. surged. In 1998 alone, sales of single herbal medicines grew by 183.2 percent ($286.5 million) in grocery, drug, and mass merchandise stores (AC Nielsen Scan Track: Spencer Information Services, 1999). The top three herbal products that increased in sales in 1999 were soy, flax, and black cohosh (Blumenthal, 2000). And although statistics suggest that herb sales have now leveled off in mainstream stores (Blumenthal, 2000), American consumers are reportedly spending up to $5.1 billion on herbal products annually (Eisenberg et al., 1998). Since the passage of the Dietary Supplement Health and Education Act of 1994, herb sales have surpassed vitamin sales.

An article published in the *Journal of the American Medical Association* reported that almost 1 in 5 adults who reported regular use of prescription drugs stated that they also used at least one herbal remedy, a vitamin supplement, or both, at the same time as their prescription medication (Eisenberg et al., 1998). In a 1999 *Prevention* magazine telephone survey of 2000 adults conducted by Princeton Survey Research Associates, 49 percent of respondents said that they had used an herbal remedy within the past year, and 24 percent reported regular use of an herbal remedy (*Prevention*, April–May 1999). Most consumers used garlic, ginseng, ginkgo, or St. John's wort, followed by echinacea. A majority (75%) said they did so to ensure good health (*Prevention*, April–May 1999). In a 1999 telephone survey of 1003 Canadians, more than two-thirds stated that natural herbal supplements are as effective as prescription drugs or over-the-counter remedies (from Traditional Medicinals Gallup Survey, 1999).

Clearly, this modern resurgence in the use of herbal medicines—and the tendency

8

of consumers to combine herbal, prescription, and over-the-counter medicines—gives health-care professionals once again the responsibility to learn about herbal medicines, routinely talk with patients about them, and take steps to guide patients appropriately.

chapter two

ARE HERBAL MEDICINES SAFE AND EFFECTIVE?

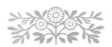

Today many consumers believe that herbal medicines are safe because they are more "natural" than prescription drugs. Added to this perception is the notion that herbs must be safe if the government deems it unnecessary to regulate herbal products under the same strict guidelines as prescription drugs. However, the fact is that government agencies have been weighing various aspects of herbal safety and regulation for many years. In 1958, under the food additive amendment to Food and Drug Administration (FDA) statutes, about 250 herbs were approved as food additives. Among them were benzoin, chamomile, dandelion, elecampane, horehound, and marshmallow root. These herbs were labeled Generally Recognized as Safe (GRAS) because of their long history of safe use. However, no category was established to judge the safe use of plants for medicinal purposes (Griggs, 1981).

In 1962, an amendment to the Federal Food, Drug, and Cosmetic Act (the Kefauver-Harris Amendment) required that medications be proved not only safe but also effective (Tyler, 1993). The FDA set up 17 panels to review the efficacy of active ingredients in all over-the-counter medications. To demonstrate efficacy, the panels used in vitro tests and complex human clinical trials. They rejected testimonials as proof of safety or efficacy. Many herbal products being used at that time were not considered medications and thus were not included in this wide-ranging investigation of safety and efficacy. In fact, only aloe, capsicum, cascara, psyllium seed and husk, senna, slippery elm, and witch hazel have been approved in the U.S. for medicinal purposes (Youngkin & Israel, 1996). Consequently, the safety and efficacy of many herbal products have been difficult to gauge—particularly given their widespread manufacturing problems. Even so, consumers have spoken out loudly against increased government regulation.

In 1993, when the FDA threatened to remove herbal products from the shelves of health food stores, Americans united in writing letters of protest. In fact, Congress received more mail of protest on this matter than on any other issue since the Vietnam War (Brevoort, 1996; Tyler, 1996). As a result, the legislators passed the Dietary Supplement Health and Education Act of 1994. Congress placed herbal medicines in the category of dietary supplements and stated, "There may be a positive relationship between sound dietary practice and good health ... although further scientific research is needed, there may be a connection between dietary supplement use, reduced health-

10

care expenses, and disease prevention." A stipulation was added that no therapeutic claims, meaning "claims relating to the diagnosis treatment, cure, or prevention of any disease," could be made on the labels of any of these products. Product labels may make "statements of nutritional support" and "structure and function." They were barred from including a disease state in the name of the product (Israelson & Blumenthal, 2000).

In 1996, President Clinton set up a Commission on Dietary Supplement Labels (CDSL). Seven herbal experts were appointed to serve on this commission. Their mission was to make dietary supplement labels informative as to health benefit claims while also promoting the safety and quality of these products and procedures for evaluating their health benefit claims (*Herb Research News,* 1996). Its final report was issued in October 1997 and concluded that:

- The supplement industry must ensure the safety of herbal medicines.
- There should be a botanical ingredient review panel.
- Incentives should exist to research herbal products.
- Traditional uses should receive approval.
- Specific guidelines should be included in new products that state the product's purpose, vendor information, product identification, ingredients (including the Latin name and plant part used), intended use, dosage, and contraindications (McCaleb & Blumenthal, 1997).

These recommendations are available on the Internet at *http://web.health.gov/dietsupp.*

MANUFACTURING PROBLEMS

Historically, one of the most difficult problems in determining the safety and efficacy of herbal products has concerned manufacturing. In past years, herbal medicines have had substantial manufacturing difficulties that have affected their safety and efficacy. They have had poor quality control. Labeling has sometimes been deceptive. They have had little standardization and very little research to substantiate their use. Some have been adulterated or contaminated with toxic metals. One incident of adulteration occurred in the summer of 1997, when a plantain product was found to be adulterated by foxglove, the plant from which digitalis is isolated (Blumenthal, 1997). In other examples, skullcap has been adulterated by germander and Siberian ginseng root has been adulterated by *Periploca sepium* root (McGuffin, 2000). Some herbal medicines imported from China have contained diazepam, camphor, and mercury. Contamination has also been caused by pesticides, molds, and excreta.

Even if a product is uncontaminated, its potency may differ from one manufacturer to another. When working with herbal products even in today's market, it is important to look for standardized extracts, which means that each dose of the product contains the same potency of herbal compounds. It is also important to always use the same product.

Today the safety of herbal products is the responsibility of each manufacturer and is regulated under Good Manufacturing Practices, which include potency, cleanliness, and stability (Soller, 2000). And although herbal supplements are not regulated in the same manner as prescription drugs, the FDA and the Federal Trade

Commission (FTC) do oversee their safety. The FDA has the power to stop the sale of a dietary supplement that is toxic (Soller, 2000), and FDA's MedWatch program tracks complaints about herbal products and logs reports of side effects caused by herbs (Love, 1998). Complaints and side effects may be reported by calling MedWatch at 800-332-1088.

The FTC, which monitors advertising claims for dietary supplements (including herbs) has also published guidelines for herbal products. Under these guidelines, herbal claims must be substantiated or the FTC can ban the claim as a false advertisement. Complaints of false claims can be made by calling 877-382-4357 (FTC-HELP) (Soller, 2000).

Regulations issued by the FDA on January 6, 2000, pertaining to dietary supplements and their claims for structure and function are available on the Internet at *www.fda.gov/OHRMS/DOCKETS/98fr/oc99257.pdf.*

RESEARCHING SAFETY

Further complicating the process of determining safety and efficacy is the fact that different nations use different criteria. Some require the results of research as the basis for claims of safety and efficacy, whereas others do not. In 1974 and 1978 the World Health Organization (WHO), UNICEF, and the Third-First World Health Assembly urged all Third-World countries to develop their own traditional medicine systems, in which no restrictions would be placed on herbal products that had been used traditionally without harm (Akerele, 1992). Despite this endorsement of traditional use by the WHO, however, an FDA spokesperson quoted in the *Journal of the American Medical Association (JAMA)* maintained that "the randomized controlled trial is still the best and, in general, the only credible source of evidence for the efficacy of most therapies." (Marwick, 1995, p. 608).

Many European studies have focused on herbal products. Some of these studies are now being replicated in the U.S. However, a direct comparison of results can be difficult because Europe and the U.S. commonly use different herbal forms. For instance, echinacea is given parenterally in Europe but is available only in tincture, tea, and capsule form in the U.S.

Germany has incorporated phytomedicines (plant medicines) into their health-care system by continuing to teach pharmacognosy in their medical schools. Medical schools commonly have botanical gardens to be used for research. German scientists research the use of standardized semipurified (still containing multiple individual chemicals) extracts to prove the safety and efficacy of their more commonly used herbs. In 1978, an expert panel of medical, pharmacy, and research scientists was convened to form the German Commission E to research the validity of herbal medicines. Monographs have now been published by the German Federal Health Agency through the German Commission E, which reviewed 380 herbs and combinations and found them to have favorable benefit:risk ratios. A monograph pertains to a single botanical medicine or a fixed combination of botanicals. These monographs have been translated by the American Botanical Council and may be purchased.

In Germany, many herbal teas and herbal products can be found standardized in pharmacies, where pharmacists give recommendations for the use of these phytomedicines. Their cost is reimbursable by health insurance companies. According to *JAMA*, "Total sales of nonprescription drugs in Germany—the largest market—in 1993 amounted to $7 billion, half prescribed and half purchased by consumers for self-medication. Of this amount, $1.9 billion was spent exclusively on plant-based medicines." By 1995, about 7 percent of drugs covered by German health insurance were herbal medicines. In Germany, these medicines are primarily being used to treat heart disease and disorders of the respiratory and gastrointestinal tracts (Marwick, 1995). Dr. Melville Eaves, business manager of Dr. Willmar Schwabe GmbH and Company, Karlsruhe, Germany (Marwick, 1995, p. 607) states that "mainstream manufacturers . . . have sought and managed to obtain many patents in this area." This last statement is very important because U.S. manufacturers have always used lack of patent protection as one of the reasons why clinical trials are not being done in the U.S.

A panel of experts in Europe has set up the European Scientific Cooperative of Phytotherapy (ESCOP) and published monographs similar to those of the German Commission E. Their goal is to encourage standardization and consistency in the use of herbal medicines in European countries. In October 1998, an international symposium was held by ESCOP to discuss European regulation of herbal medicines. Some countries have very strict controls on the safety and efficacy of herbal medicines; in other countries, the use of herbal medicines stems solely from traditional use. ESCOP has published 60 monographs with 15 herb-drug interactions, many with the same interactions noted by the German Commission E (Blumenthal, 2000).

Internationally, the WHO is trying to develop monographs, assess the safety and efficacy of herbal medicines, protect plants for medicinal use, and protect consumers through quality control standards (Upton, 1999). The first volume, published in 1999, included 28 herbs; the second volume was scheduled to include 30 herbs.

According to Upton (1999, p. 59), "The *United States Pharmacopeia* has issued standard monographs for chamomile, feverfew, ginger, ginger powder, garlic, powdered garlic, ginseng, and ginseng powder. Proposed monographs include hawthorn, hawthorn powder, milk thistle, powdered milk thistle, valerian, and a monograph on extracts in general. Monographs currently in progress include echinacea purpurea, ginkgo, and St. John's wort."

Even though the U.S. seems to be lagging in the practice of herbal medicine, it is making strides in recognizing the need for more research in this area. By congressional mandate in 1992, the National Institutes of Health (NIH) established the Office of Alternative Medicine to evaluate and establish grants for research into alternative medicine, including herbal medicine (Weisman, 1994). In 1999, the National Cancer Institute (NCI) established its own Office of Cancer Complementary and Alternative Medicine, which is already supporting clinical trials on herbal medicines such as green tea and their benefits in cancer treatment. NCI's website (nccam.nih.gov). Today the Office of Alternative Medicine is now called the National Center for Complementary and Alternative Medicine (NCCAM) and has a budget of almost $70 million.

13

chapter three

THE ROLE OF HEALTH-CARE PROFESSIONALS IN HERBAL MEDICINE

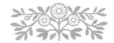

With the increase in the use of herbal medicines and the continuing evolution of product regulation, health-care practitioners must be open and unbiased about these increasingly popular products. Although some patients resist telling primary care providers about their use of herbal medicine, others do discuss it. However, if the provider responds with the blanket assertion that herbal medicines are harmful, unsafe, and unproven, the patient not only becomes frightened and discouraged but also is less likely to talk about herb use with other health-care professionals. Naturally, this approach raises risks for patients and harms the relationship between patient and provider. If a patient takes an herb that interacts with a prescribed drug, the results could be disastrous.

Consequently, it is imperative that health-care professionals educate themselves about herbal medicines in general, including the possibility of herb-drug interactions, or that they consider referring patients who wish to take herbal remedies to an herbalist. The first and foremost priority is taking an accurate history and asking specific questions about herbal medicines and foods that a patient consumes daily, especially in large amounts, that may interact with conventional medicines. Some of the herbs patients may consume daily in large amounts are coffee, ginseng, chamomile, garlic, ginger, turmeric, and peppermint.

Patients need to be warned about experimenting with herbal medicines, especially if they are seeing multiple health-care providers, one or more of whom may be unaware of all the herbs and medicines the patient is taking. Persons who are at risk for adverse reactions should make sure their herbal source is reliable. If patients are known to have adverse drug reactions, allergies, chronic skin rashes, or pre-existing liver disease from conventional medicines, they should be warned about the increased risk of adverse effects from taking herbs. Elderly patients, pregnant women, and children also have increased risk of developing problems while taking herbal medicines.

Health-care providers who recommend herbal medicines for specific conditions should encourage patients to purchase standardized herbal products from a single company to help ensure the potency of the desired plant compound. Patients should be encouraged to "purchase products that list the herb name, the concentration of its active constituents, an expiration date, the manufacturer's name and contact information" (Ramsey et al., 2000; Bauer, 2000). Bauer (2000) also suggests looking for the *U.S. Pharmacopeia* (*USP*) or *National Formulary* (*NF*) symbols to help determine the quality of the product.

Finally, health-care providers who recommend herbal medicines should adopt certain legal considerations, such as those that follow:

- Become educated in herbal medicine by attending workshops, courses, and conferences.
- Contact companies who make herbal preparations and investigate how their products are harvested or obtained, dried, and manufactured.
- Keep at least one clinical trial on file for each herbal remedy you choose to recommend to a patient.
- Recommend only herbal remedies of which you have knowledge.
- Consider having the patient sign a consent form that outlines your recommendation for an herbal medicine instead of or in addition to a conventional treatment plan.
- Include in each patient's history direct questions about the use of complementary therapies, especially questions on the use of herbal medicines. Be unbiased and know that it takes time to develop trust between you and your patient.
- Caution patients not to experiment with herbal medicines, especially when they have more than one health-care provider who may not be aware of all the drugs the patient is taking.
- If you know that a patient has adverse drug reactions, allergies, chronic skin rashes, or pre-existing liver disease from conventional medicines, warn the patient about the increased risk of side effects from herbs and the importance of reporting any side effects (of conventional drugs or herbs) to the primary care provider. Also, warn elderly patients, pregnant women, and children that they have an increased risk of adverse effects from herbal medicines.
- Keep a referral list of knowledgeable herbalists.
- Tell patients to make sure their herbal source is reliable. The active constituents of the herbal product should be listed on the label. Recommend herbal products that have been standardized to the German Commission E requirements and may also contain the letters USP or NF.
- Urge patients to take only the recommended dosages of herbal medicines and discourage them from taking herbal products on a daily, long-term basis. If long-term use is needed for a chronic illness, recommend occasional breaks in therapy. You or the patient should consult with a knowledgeable herbalist about long-term use.
- Caution patients to be especially careful when considering herbal therapy during pregnancy or breast-feeding. Again, consider referring the patient to an herbalist or other knowledgeable clinician who specializes in the health of women and children.

chapter four

FROM HERB TO MEDICINE: FORMS OF HERBAL PRODUCTS

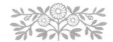

Obviously, herbal products start as plants. They make the journey from plant to medicine by being either harvested from the wild (called wild-crafting) or grown for the purpose of creating an herbal medicine. Keep in mind that many herbs are endangered in the wild from either overuse or destruction of habitat. Some of the herbs that are currently at risk in the wild include American ginseng, black cohosh, bloodroot, blue cohosh, echinacea, goldenseal, helonias root, kava kava, lady's slipper orchid, osha, partridge berry, peyote, slippery elm, sundew, trillium bethroot, true unicorn, Venus's flytrap, and wild yam.

If you wish to work with herbs, don't search in the wild to obtain them. Instead, create an herb garden and grow and harvest the herbs yourself. After harvesting an herb, dry it to reduce the moisture content without destroying the plant's active chemical compounds. The herb should be dried by spreading it loosely on a rack so that air can circulate around it to prevent mold. The procedure for harvesting and preparing each herb varies with the time of year and the part of the plant that will be used for medicinal purposes. Herbs should be stored in dark glass containers with tight-fitting lids, away from sunlight and heat.

Besides the tablets, capsules, syrups, and lozenges that may be available commercially, common forms of herbal products include teas, tinctures, extracts, and external forms.

HERBAL TEAS (WATER-BASED EXTRACTS)

In China, herbal teas are prescribed by practitioners for specific illnesses and are made from about 12 different herbs, all of them balancing and complementing each other to prevent side effects. The practitioner gives the patient a bag of medicinal leaves, roots, and other substances and tells the patient to add water, simmer like a soup, and drink as directed throughout the day. Herbal teas are gaining popularity here in the United States. You can now find them in health food stores, grocery stores, and restaurants. You can make your own tea bags by placing 1 teaspoon of dried herb into a tea bag and then sealing it with a hot iron. Or you can prepare teas using a tea ball, tea strainer, or prepared tea bags.

For an adult, the usual recommended dose of tea is one teacupful. For an acute condition the patient may drink small amounts of tea more often, up to three cups a day. Chronic conditions may warrant three cups a day as well. For a child, the dosage may be calculated by using Young's rule (for children age 2 and over) or Clark's rule as shown below.

$$\text{Young's rule: } \frac{\text{Age (in years)}}{\text{Age (in years)} \times 12} \times \text{Adult dose} = \text{Child's dose}$$

$$\text{Clark's rule: } \frac{\text{Weight (lb)}}{150} \times \text{Adult dose} = \text{Child's dose}$$

If a mother is breast-feeding and would like to administer an herbal remedy to her infant, the dose would be for the mother to drink 1 teacupful and then breast-feed her infant. The herb will be transmitted through the breast milk. If preferred, cooled tea may be administered by a dropperful directly into the baby's mouth. Different herbs should be taken for differing lengths of time.

Herbal Tea Infusion

An herbal infusion refers to an herbal preparation in which water is used as the solvent to extract the chemical compounds of the herbal medicine into the water. It is then taken internally. Fresh herbs are best for preparing herbal teas. Generally, three parts of fresh herbs are equal to one part of dried herb. So, if one teaspoonful of dried tea is recommended, three teaspoonfuls of herb may be substituted. An infusion uses the herb's flowers, seeds, leafy parts, or roots that contain volatile oils (examples are valerian root and goldenseal root). Prepare them by steeping the plant parts in water, creating a concentrated herbal tea.

For a hot herbal tea infusion, bring fresh, cool water to a boil in a pot. In general, glass, enamel, stainless steel, or cast iron pots are preferred. Use 1 teaspoonful of dried herb to 8 ounces of boiling water. Let the herb sit and brew for about 10 minutes, strain, and cool. Examples of herbs to use in an infusion are chamomile, nettles, fever-few, and peppermint. (Always cover the cup when brewing peppermint tea to preserve the volatile oils.) For a cold herbal tea infusion (sun tea), place three tablespoons of herb and one quart of water in a glass jar and cover with a lid. Place in a sunny window for several hours, and voilà! Strain and you'll have a delicious tea.

Refrigerate any unused portions of herb tea. Infusions are not easily preserved and need to be kept refrigerated and used within a day or two.

Decoction

A decoction is similar to an infusion, but it is used to brew the roots, barks, nonaromatic seeds, and twigs of plants. Bring fresh, cool water to boil in a nonmetal pot. Use 1 level teaspoon of roots, barks, twigs, or seeds to 8 ounces of water. Cover with a lid, bring to a boil, and simmer for 15 to 20 minutes. Then strain and cool.

Examples of herbs that can be used in a decoction are black cohosh root and kava kava root. Valerian root and goldenseal root should be infused rather than prepared as a decoction because of their volatile oils.

Refrigerate any unused portions. Decoctions are not well preserved and need to be kept refrigerated and used within a day or two.

TINCTURES

A tincture is a concentrated herbal extract made by soaking an herb in alcohol, vinegar, or glycerine. The solvent extracts the chemical compounds of the herb. Tinctures are sold in small, dark bottles, usually 1 to 4 ounces, and are tightly closed with a dropper. A 1:5 ratio on the label means that the tincture contains 1 part herb (weighing one gram) to 5 parts (5 grams) of extract. Milliliters (mL) are used in dosages, and one mL is equal to one gram. One dropperful of a 1:5 extract means that five dropperfuls will be needed to get the dosage of 1 gram of herb. Tinctures may be used internally or externally.

Alcohol is the most commonly used of the three solvents. It extracts the active compounds of the plant, concentrates the herb, and acts as a great preservative. Commercial tinctures use ethyl alcohol. The herb's active compounds are then extracted, and the alcohol acts as a preservative. The shelf-life of a tincture is from 3 to 10 years. Full-strength apple cider vinegar may be used also; it has a shelf life of 1 to 2 years.

Vegetable glycerine may also be used as a solvent to extract the active compounds of the herb. Glycerine is a better choice for those who prefer not to ingest alcohol, for diabetics, and for children. Glycerine is processed in the body as a fat, not a sugar, even though it has a sweet taste on the tongue. One caution is that if more than one ounce of glycerine is taken, it may cause a laxative effect. Glycerine is generally diluted with 50 percent distilled water. A small percentage of alcohol (5% to 10%) may be added to increase shelf-life. When glycerine is used as a solvent, the shelf-life is only about 6 months to 2 years. Glycerine should not be the solvent of choice for herbs that contain resins and gums; alcohol is needed to properly extract the active constituents of these herbs. Glycerine tinctures should be refrigerated for best effects.

Examples of herbs suitable for tincture are dandelion, valerian, St. John's wort, peppermint, black cohosh, and chaste tree berry. Tinctures may be diluted in juice or water or placed directly on the tongue. Dosages are usually given by dropperfuls and vary in size. For an acute condition, such as a cold, 1 dose can be given every 2 to 4 hours. For chronic conditions, doses are given less frequently and need to be monitored by a health-care practitioner. If a patient is unable to take a tincture orally, it may be rubbed on the abdomen at three times the normal dose. It may also be added to the bath at about 10 to 20 times the oral dose.

Making Your Own Herbal Tincture

To make a tincture with dried herbs, fill a sterilized canning jar with finely chopped dried herb, leaving 2 inches of space between the herb and the top of the jar. (Or use one part herb to five parts solvent.) Pour solvent (usually vodka) into the jar until it covers the herb. Don't let any of the plant parts extend above the solvent or they may become moldy. Label and date the jar and place it in a dark place at room temperature. Shake it daily. After about 6 weeks, strain the liquid through cheesecloth and squeeze out the residue. Place the tincture in small, dark tincture bottles, then label and date them.

You may also blend herbs and solvent in the blender and then place the resulting liquid into a wide-mouthed jar. For fresh herbs, the ratio is one part herb to two parts solvent because of the high water content of fresh herbs. Then follow the directions given previously.

EXTRACTS

Extracts come in three forms: fluidextracts, solid extracts, and standardized extracts. Fluidextracts use vinegar, glycerine, or glycol as a solvent and are more concentrated than tinctures. When herbal extracts are made commercially, more complicated methods of distillation are used at lower temperatures. During this process, some of the beneficial compounds of the whole plant (such as fiber) are discarded, leaving only the active constituent(s) to be standardized.

Solid extracts are extremely concentrated because the solvent is completely removed, leaving a soft solid or dry solid extract. The dry solid extract can be ground into a coarse or fine powder. During this process, as with fluidextracts, some of the beneficial compounds of the whole plant (such as fiber) are discarded, leaving only the active constituent(s) to be standardized. A fluidextract or tincture can then be made by diluting a solid extract with water or alcohol.

Standardized extracts are those that contain consistent amounts of specific plant compounds responsible for the plant's health benefits. This standardized form is sold in Germany and is beginning to be sold in the United States. An example of an herb with standardized active chemical compounds is kava kava. The problem is that some of the chemical compounds responsible for health benefits are unknown in some herbs. In this case, marker compounds are used. Marker compounds are those that are found in the highest amount in the herb and are thought to have the greatest effect. Valerian is an example of an herb in which the specific chemical compound is unknown. The other problem with standardized extracts is that herbal potency varies among manufacturers' products.

EXTERNAL FORMS

External forms for application of herbs include herbal baths, oils, salves, ointments, poultices, compresses, and liniments.

Herbal Baths

Place about 6 ounces of dried or fresh herb in a small muslin sack and let it float in the bathtub while you are bathing. A tincture, decoction, or infusion may also be added to the bath at about 10 times the dose you would take by mouth. Examples of herbs to use in the bath are yarrow heads for fever (let them float freely) and chamomile, lavender, and rose petals for relaxation.

Herbal Oils

These products may be used for massages or to heal dry skin. Place 2 cups of olive, safflower, or canola oil in a glass or an enameled double boiler. Then place 3 ounces of herb—single or in combination—in the pot and simmer for up to 30 minutes. Do not boil; if you see the entire mixture bubbling or smoking, the oil is too hot. Afterward, strain and pour into small jars. For a calming, relaxing oil, use 1 ounce each of lavender flowers, rose petals, and chamomile flowers. For dry skin, use 2 cups of canola oil and 3 ounces of calendula flowers.

To make an herbal massage oil infusion, pick the herb, dry it overnight, and place it in a clean container. Cover it with extra virgin olive oil (thicker than other oils) or almond, sunflower, or safflower oil. Make sure that none of the plant parts extend above the oil or your oil will become moldy. Let the container sit in a sunny, warm window for about 2 weeks. Then strain and place the oil in pretty jars. An excellent herb for this type of oil is St. John's wort. Pick the buds when the leaves are dotted with red spots. Your fingers will turn red as you pick them. Place the buds gently into a container and cover with oil. Place in a sunny spot and, in about 2 weeks, the oil will turn red. Strain it and use as a massage oil all winter for any type of strain, sprain, backache, or sports injury.

Herbal Salves

Herbal salves are used primarily for dry skin and healing of superficial wounds. To make a salve, place 1/4 cup of beeswax into the top of a double boiler. As the beeswax melts, add 1 cup of herbal oil, stir, and cool. Pour into small salve jars. Label and date the jars, and refrigerate them for shelf life.

Caution patients not to use herbal salves for deep or infected wounds. Tell them that signs of infection include redness, drainage, warmth in the area, and tenderness. Urge patients to contact a health-care practitioner immediately if the area looks infected or does not begin to heal within a few days.

For chapped lips or cold sores, consider making a lip balm by adding more beeswax than you would in a normal salve. The added beeswax increases the hardness of the salve. Red raspberry leaves and lemon balm are two herbs that are helpful for cold sores.

Herbal Ointments

Herbal ointments are also used topically for superficial wound healing. Add 3 ounces of herb to about 6 ounces of petroleum or nonpetroleum jelly. Let them simmer but not boil. Remove from heat, strain the herb using cheesecloth, and place in small jars. Label and date. Store in a cool, dark place. Ointments should last up to a month or longer. Examples of herbs that are great to use in ointment form are calendula for superficial wound healing, eczema and diaper rash; goldenseal for cuts to prevent infection, and comfrey for superficial wound healing. Do not use herbal ointments for deep wounds. Signs of infection include redness, drainage, warmth in the area, and soreness. If area looks infected, or does not begin to heal within a few days, please consult your health-care practitioner immediately.

Poultices

A poultice is used externally to relax muscles or to ease minor skin eruptions, poison ivy, insect bites, superficial wounds, and inflammation. To make a poultice, mash fresh herbs in hot water and wrap the plant part in gauze. Cool it until it can be safely applied to the skin, then apply it to the affected area. Poultices may be applied up to three times a day. They can be made using:

- Goldenseal, which has astringent properties that are useful for infections. Make powder into a paste by mixing with warm water.
- Plantain (use fresh and apply directly to bee stings).
- Jewelweed (wonderful for poison ivy relief when used as a poultice or compress).
- Comfrey (helpful for superficial wounds and hemorrhoids when used as a poultice or compress.

Compresses

Compresses are used externally and can be either warm or cold. Cold compresses reduce inflammation and help to relieve pain. They are used initially for sprains, contusions, strains, inflammation, headaches, and insect bites. Warm compresses are used to increase circulation to an area and to allow muscles, tendons, and ligaments to stretch. Warm compresses may be used for poison ivy also.

For a warm compress, prepare an infusion of herbs in hot water and then dip gauze or a cotton cloth into the infusion at the desired temperature and apply the cloth to the area. Or you can dilute a tincture in warm or cold water and then soak a cloth in the solution. Examples of herbs used for compresses include ginger (a warming, stimulating herb used to relieve inflammation) and cayenne (a stimulating herb that is excellent for muscle aches).

Liniments

Liniments are for external use for aches and pains. Prepare the liniment the same way as you would a tincture, but use rubbing alcohol, witch hazel, or vinegar as the solvent. Place the herb(s) in a canning jar and cover with the solvent. Place the jar in a warm, dark area and shake it every day for 2 weeks. Strain it and store the liniment in dark bottles. Label and date the bottles.

Examples of herbs commonly used in liniments include yarrow leaf, wintergreen leaves, cayenne, plantain leaf, rosemary leaves, and yellow dock leaf and root. Do not use liniments on cuts or broken skin.

21

part 2

HERBS

INTRODUCTION

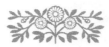

Each of the herbs included in this book is presented in the following format for convenience and ease of use. The patient teaching information provided for each herb uses a similar but simpler format. These pages can be photocopied for distribution to patients.

Historical Uses

This section recounts how the herb has been used historically or described in folklore.

Growth

Here you will find brief information on where the plant can be found or how it is grown.

Part(s) Used

This section describes the part or parts of the herb that are used for medicinal effects.

Major Chemical Compound(s)

This section lists important chemical compounds that are present in the herb. All herbal medicines are made up of chemical compounds that explain the characteristics of the herb, including its mechanism of action, taste, intended effects, and side effects. The following is a list of some of the compounds that you will encounter when using herbs, along with a brief description of each compound's effects.

- Acids: antiseptic and cleansing properties
- Alkaloids: effects on the central nervous system that are sometimes toxic and addictive
- Anthraquinones: irritating and laxative effects
- Bitters: acts to improve digestion
- Coumarins: anticoagulant (blood-thinning) properties
- Flavones: anti-inflammatory, anti-spasmodic, sometimes diuretic effects
- Glycosides: include cardiac glycosides (which affect the heart), cyanogenic glycosides (which have antispasmodic and sedative effects and alter heart rate), mustard oil (which is very irritating), and sulfur (which has antibiotic properties)
- Mucilages: slimy and soothing to mucous membranes
- Resins: astringent, antiseptic effects

- Saponins: anti-inflammatory (chemically resemble steroidal hormones) and produce a lather in water
- Tannins: antiseptic, astringent effects
- Volatile oils: antiseptic, stimulant effects

Clinical Uses

In this section you will find a brief description of how the herb is typically used.

Mechanism of Action

This section explains our current understanding of the herb's pharmacological actions, which typically result from the chemical compounds it contains.

Dosage

Here you will find suggested dosages of the herb in the form of teas, tinctures, salves, ointments, and oils and how often they should be taken or applied.

Side Effects

Like traditional drugs, herbs may have adverse effects. These unwanted effects are described in this section.

Contraindications

In this section you will find warnings for persons who should not take the herb and circumstances in which the herb should not be used.

Herb-Drug Interactions

This section describes prescription drugs with which the herb should not be taken.

Pregnancy and Breast-Feeding

Here you will find safety recommendations for women who are pregnant or breast-feeding.

Pediatric Patients

Used only when appropriate, this section describes special considerations for children.

SUMMARY OF STUDIES

Selected supportive clinical studies, when available, are described in this section.

REFERENCES

Sources used to provide information for each herb are given for each herb entry.

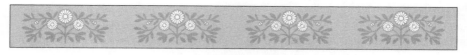

ALOE
(Aloe vera)

Historical Uses

Aloe has been used as a medicinal plant to heal the skin for more than 4000 years. It is also called the burn plant.

Growth

This member of the lily family may grow to 30 feet or more in height. It may also be grown as a houseplant and is cultivated in the West Indies. Unlike most plants, aloe may be grown in the bedroom because it may be beneficial, helping to increase oxygen during sleep time and removing toxins (Wood, 1999).

Part Used

• Gel inside leaves

Major Chemical Compounds

• Anthraquinones (aloin, barbaloin)
• Polysaccharides (glycoproteins, acemannan, mucopolysaccharides)
• Prostaglandins
• Fatty acids
• Zinc
• Vitamins C and E

Clinical Uses

Aloe is discussed here for external use only. It may be applied topically for wound healing, insect bites, burns, and sunburn.

Mechanism of Action

Prostaglandins decrease inflammation and promote wound healing. Vitamin C, vitamin E, and zinc are needed for wound healing also. Polysaccharides assist in wound repair and epidermal growth.

Dosage

In the store, look for products that list aloe as the first ingredient. Apply aloe vera gel liberally to wounds or burns. If using a leaf from an aloe plant, wash the leaf thoroughly, snip off a piece, open the leaf, and scrape away some of the gel. Then apply the gel directly to the wound. Refrigerate any leftover gel to keep it from spoiling.

Side Effects

None are known.

Contraindications

- Do not apply to deep wounds.
- Aloe may delay surgical wound healing after a laparotomy (Tyler, 1994).

Herb-Drug Interactions

None are known.

Pregnancy and Breast-Feeding

Aloe may delay surgical wound healing after a Caesarean section (Tyler, 1994).

Pediatric Patients

No restrictions are known.

SUMMARY OF STUDIES

Roberts & Travis (*1995*). In a study of wound healing in mice, aloe gel applied daily for 2 weeks reduced acute radiation-induced skin reactions in mice, whereas lubricating jelly and healing ointment did not.

Davis et al. (*1994*). In an assay using saline controls in wound healing in mice, aloe improved wound healing and inhibited inflammation.

Davis et al. (*1994*). In a wound tensile strength assay in mice, aloe vera at 100 and 300 mg/kg daily for 4 days blocked the wound-healing suppression of hydrocortisone acetate up to 100 percent using the assay. There was a dose-response relationship.

Davis et al. (*1992*). In this in vivo study, aloe vera inhibited inflammation, stimulated fibroblasts, and promoted wound healing without side effects.

REFERENCES

Davis, R., DiDonato, J., Hartman, G., & Haas, R. (1994). Anti-inflammatory and wound healing activity of a growth substance in *Aloe vera*. *Journal of the American Podiatric Medical Association, 84,* 77–81.

Davis, R., DiDonato, J., Johnson, R., & Stewart, C. (1994). *Aloe vera,* hydrocortisone, and sterol influence on wound tensile strength and anti-inflammation. *Journal of the American Podiatric Medical Association, 84,* 614–621.

Davis, R., Stewart, G., & Bregman, P. (1992). Aloe vera and the inflamed synovial pouch model. *Journal of the American Podiatric Medical Association, 82,* 140–148.

Roberts, D., & Travis, E. (1995). Acemannan-containing wound dressing gel reduces radiation-induced skin reactions in C3H mice. *International Journal of Radiation Oncology, Biology, Physics, 32,* 1047–1052.

Tyler, V. (1994). *Herbs of choice.* Binghamton, NY: Pharmaceutical Products Press.

Wood, R. (1999). *The new whole foods encyclopedia.* New York: Penguin.

NOTES

NOTES

ALOE
(Aloe vera)

Historical Uses

Aloe has been used as a medicinal plant to heal the skin for more than 4000 years. It is also known as the burn plant.

Growth

This member of the lily family may grow to be 30 feet or more in height. It may be grown as a houseplant and is cultivated in the West Indies. Unlike most plants, aloe may be kept in the bedroom because it may have beneficial effects, increasing oxygen while you sleep and removing toxins.

Part Used

• Gel inside leaves

Medical Uses

Aloe is discussed here for external use only. It may be applied topically for wound healing, insect bites, burns, and sunburn.

Dosage

In the store, look for products that list aloe as the first ingredient. Apply aloe vera gel liberally to wounds or burns. If using a leaf from an aloe plant at home, wash the leaf thoroughly, snip off a piece, open the leaf, and scrape away some of the gel. Then apply the gel directly to the wound. Refrigerate any leftover gel to keep it from spoiling.

Warnings

• Don't apply aloe to deep wounds. It may delay wound healing after a laparotomy or a Caesarean section.
• No restrictions are known during breast-feeding.
• No restrictions are known for children.

31

BILBERRY
(Vaccinium myrtillus)

Historical Uses

This herb has been used since the Middle Ages, primarily in Europe, for kidney disorders, diarrhea, respiratory infections, and treatment for scurvy (McCaleb et al., 2000).

Growth

Bilberry is known as the European blueberry and is larger than the American blueberry. It grows in temperate zones. Bilberry and blueberry are from the same family.

Parts Used

- Dried, ripe fruit
- Leaves

Major Chemical Compounds

- Glucoquinones (in leaves), which reduce blood glucose
- Anthocyanosides (in fruits), which have been shown experimentally to dilate blood vessels
- Tannins, flavonoids (Bown, 1995)

Clinical Uses

Bilberry is used for antioxidant effects and for varicose veins, night blindness, diabetes, diarrhea, hemorrhoids, and gum inflammation (Bown, 1995). It is approved by the German Commission E for "non-specific acute diarrhea, mild inflammation of the mucous membranes and throat" (Blumenthal et al., 2000). It may be used to treat non-specific diarrhea in children, as noted in Blumenthal et al. (2000).

Mechanism of Action

The tannins in the bilberry fruit have astringent properties that are helpful in easing diarrhea. Bilberry fruits also contain anthocyanosides, which are helpful because of their antioxidant effects, for forming collagen in connective tissue around blood vessels, and for eye health. Anthocyanosides have been shown to be helpful in preventing the breakdown and promoting the regeneration of rhodopsin in the rods of the retina (Blumenthal et al., 2000; McCaleb et al., 2000). Bilberry leaves contain glucoquinones, which may reduce blood glucose.

Dosage

Dry extract: 80 to 160 mg standardized to 25 percent anthocyanosides two or three times a day. Take with food.

Tea: 1 teaspoon herb in 8 ounces of water, boiled for 10 minutes, then strained. For diarrhea, may use for up to 4 days.

The typical dose of bilberry extract is equal to about 3 bowls of bilberries a day (McCaleb et al., 2000).

Side Effects

Bilberry leaf may lower blood glucose and triglyceride levels.

Contraindications

Bilberry may be contraindicated in some patients because it affects clotting time by decreasing platelet aggregation.

Herb-Drug Interactions

Caution is warranted during use with anticoagulants.

Pregnancy and Breast-Feeding

No restrictions are known for bilberry fruits (Blumenthal et al., 2000). Leaves should not be used during pregnancy or breast-feeding (*Natural Medicines,* 2000)

SUMMARY OF STUDIES

No recent clinical studies in humans are available.

REFERENCES

Blumenthal, M., Goldberg, A., & Brinckmann, J. (Eds.). (2000). *Herbal medicine expanded Commission E monographs.* Austin, TX: American Botanical Council; Newton, MA: Integrative Medicine Communications.

Bown, D. (1995). *The Herb Society of America encyclopedia of herbs and their uses.* New York: Dorling Kindersley Publishing.

McCaleb, R., Leigh, E., & Morien, K. (2000). *The encyclopedia of popular herbs.* Roseville, CA: Prima Publishing.

Natural Medicines Comprehensive Database. (2000). *Pharmacist's Letter and Prescriber's Letter.* Therapeutic Research Faculty.

NOTES

BILBERRY
(Vaccinium myrtillus)

Historical Uses

This herb has been used since the Middle Ages, mainly in Europe, for kidney disorders, diarrhea, respiratory infections, and scurvy.

Growth

Known as the European blueberry, the bilberry is larger than the American blueberry. It grows in temperate zones. Bilberry and blueberry are from the same family.

Parts Used

• Dried, ripe fruit
• Leaves

Medical Uses

Bilberry is used as an antioxidant and as a treatment for varicose veins, night blindness, diabetes, diarrhea, hemorrhoids, and gum inflammation. It may be used to treat diarrhea in children.

Dosage

Dry extract: 80 to 160 mg dry extract standardized to 25 percent anthocyanosides 2 or 3 times a day. Take with food.

Tea: Place 1 teaspoon herb in 8 ounces of water, boil for 10 minutes, then strain. For diarrhea, you may use bilberry up to 4 days.

The typical dose of bilberry extract is equal to about 3 bowls of bilberries a day.

Warnings

• Bilberry leaf may lower blood glucose and triglyceride levels.
• Bilberry may affect clotting times by decreasing platelet aggregation. Use it cautiously if you take a blood thinner.
• Don't use bilberry leaves if you are pregnant or breast-feeding. No restrictions are known for the fruits.

RECIPES

BILBERRY BREAD (may substitute blueberries)

1 cup milk
1 egg
¾ cup sugar
¼ cup oil

3 teaspoons baking powder
2 cups flour
2 cups bilberries or blueberries
¼ cup molasses

Mix and spread on greased and floured cookie sheet with sides. Bake at 350° for 20 minutes.

BLUEBERRY FRUIT SMOOTHIE

1 cup low-fat blueberry yogurt
1 cup bilberries or blueberries

⅓ cup nonfat dry milk

Blend in the blender until smooth. Enjoy!

BLACK COHOSH
(Cimicifuga racemosa)

Historical Uses

In China, black cohosh root has been used for centuries for menopausal symptoms and women's health in general. Native Americans and Eclectic physicians used black cohosh for rheumatism, menstrual difficulties, and sore throats. Native American women have used it for menopausal symptoms such as hot flashes, anxiety, and depression (McKenna et al., 2001). Do not confuse it with blue cohosh.

Growth

Black cohosh is a member of the buttercup family. It is native to the northeastern U. S. and grows in sunny areas in temperate zones. An at-risk endangered herb, black cohosh can be grown in herb gardens. The roots may be harvested after 2 years.

Part Used

• Root

Major Chemical Compounds

• Triterpene
• Glycosides

Clinical Uses

Studies show that black cohosh is safe and helpful in relieving menopausal symptoms (Liske, 1998; Hardy, 2000), particularly mood swings, hot flashes, profuse sweating, and sleep disturbances (Hardy, 2000). It is "a safe, effective alternative to estrogen replacement therapy for patients who canot take estrogen replacement therapy" (Lieberman, 1998). Black cohosh may help prevent breast cancer (Dixon-Shanies & Shaikh, 1999). It has been approved by the German Commission E for "PMS, menopausal symptoms, and dysmenorrhea" (Blumenthal et al., 2000). It has been the largest-selling herbal dietary supplement for menopause in the U. S. (Blumenthal, 1998).

Mechanism of Action

Black cohosh is sometimes called a phytoestrogen. These substances are defined as "plant compounds that are structurally or functionally similar to steroidal estrogens produced by the body" (Ramsey et al., 1999, 27). A phytoestrogen has estrogen-like

37

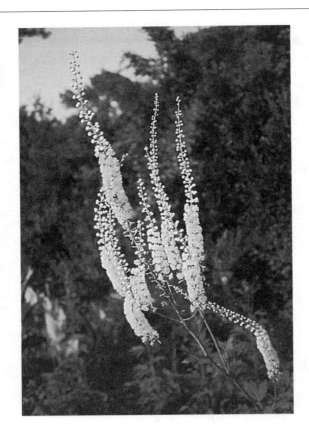

action (Liu et al., 2001) because it binds to estrogen receptors. Black cohosh suppresses luteinizing hormone (Foster, 1999; Duker et al., 1991; Stoll, 1987) with no effect on follicle-stimulating hormone (Duker et al., 1991; Stoll, 1987). It exhibits no signs of estrogenic effects in animal models and may decrease endogenous estrogen levels rather than the level of estrogenic hormones (Einer-Jensen et al., 1996).

Dosage

Tincture and tablets: 40 drops of standardized tincture or one 40-mg tablet twice daily, standardized to 4 mg triterpenes for up to 6 months.

Remifemin: The German product used in clinical studies is Remifemin, which is also distributed in the U.S. The suggested dose is 1 tablet twice a day.

Tea: For a decoction, bring 1 teaspoon of black cohosh root to a boil in 8 ounces of water, simmer about 15 minutes, strain, and drink up to 3 times a day.

Side Effects

Occasional gastrointestinal discomfort (McGuffin et al., 1997).

38

Contraindications

- Black cohosh is not recommended during pregnancy.
- It is not known whether this herb can be taken with hormone therapy.
- It is not recommended for children (McCaleb et al., 2000).

Herb-Drug Interactions

Use with hormone therapy has not been studied (Foster, 1999). The "extract augmented the anti-proliferative effect of tamoxifen" (Foster, 1999).

Pregnancy and Breast-Feeding

Do not use in pregnant women (although this herb has been used historically during labor) because it has uterine stimulant effects (McGuffin et al., 1997). In a survey of certified nursing midwives who used herbal preparations, 45 percent stated that they used black cohosh to stimulate labor (McFarlin et al., 1999).

Do not use in breast-feeding women (Blumenthal et al., 2000).

Pediatric Patients

Black cohosh is not recommended for children (McCaleb et al., 2000).

SUMMARY OF STUDIES

Stoll (1987). This randomized, double-blind, comparative, placebo-controlled study included 80 female patients over a period of 12 weeks. The study compared the effects of two tablets of black cohosh extract b.i.d. with a daily dosage of 0.625 mg conjugated estrogens and placebo. Results: Black cohosh was well tolerated and subjects showed an increase in vaginal epithelium with significant improvements in psychological symptoms not experienced with estrogen and placebo.

Duker et al. (1991). This open, controlled, comparative study involved 110 female patients at a gynecologic clinic over an 8-week period. Results: Black cohosh was related to selective LH suppression in menopausal women with no effect on follicle-stimulating hormone levels.

McKenna et al. (2001). In a review article, these investigators stated that "Remifemin was most commonly prescribed as an effective alternative to hormone replacement therapy for menopause."

Clinical studies of 1700 patients support the use of black cohosh for up to 6 months when hormone therapy is contraindicated.

Many clinical studies have been done using Remifemin with positive results (Foster, 1999; McCaleb, 2000).

REFERENCES

Blumenthal, M., Busse, W., Goldberg, A., Gruenwald, J., Hall, T., Riggins, C., & Rister, R. (Eds.). (1998). *The complete German Commission E monographs: Therapeutic guide to herbal medicines.* (S. Klein & R. Rister, Trans.). Austin, TX: American Botanical Council; Newton, MA: Integrative Medicine Communications.

Blumenthal, M., Goldberg, A., & Brinckmann, J. (Eds.). (2000). *Herbal medicine expanded Commission E monographs.* Austin, TX: American Botanical Council; Newton, MA: Integrative Medicine Communications.

Dixon-Shanties, D., & Shaikh, N. (1999). Growth inhibition of human breast cancer cells by herbs and phytoestrogens. *Oncology Reports, 6*(6), 1383–1387.

Duker, E., Kopanski, L., Jarry, H., & Wuttke, W. (1991). Effects of extracts from Cimicifuga racemosa on gonadotropin release in menopausal women and ovariectomized rats. *Planta Medica, 57,* 420–424.

Einer-Jensen, N., Zhao, J., Andersen, K., & Kristoffersen, K. (1996). *Cimicifuga* and *Melbrosia* lack oestrogenic effects in mice and rats. *Maturitas, 25,* 149–153.

Foster, S. (1999). Black cohosh: A literature review. *HerbalGram, 45,* 35–49.

Hardy, M. L. (2000). Herbs of special interest to women. *Journal of the American Pharmaceutical Association, 40*(2), 234–242.

Lieberman, S. (1998). A review of the effectiveness of *Cimicifuga racemosa* (black cohosh) for the symptoms of menopause. *Journal of Women's Health, 7*(5), 525–529.

Liske, E. (1998). Therapeutic efficacy and safety of *Cimicifuga racemosa* for gynecologic disorders. *Advances in Therapy, 15*(1), 45–53.

Liu, Z., Yang, Z., Zhu, M., & Huo, J. (2001). Estrogenicity of black cohosh (*Cimicifuga racemosa*) and its effect on estrogen receptor level in human breast cancer MCF-7 cells. *Wei Sheng Yan Jiu (Journal of Hygiene Research), 30*(2), 77–80.

McCaleb, R., Leigh, E., & Morien, K. (2000). *The encyclopedia of popular herbs.* Roseville, CA: Prima Publishing.

McFarlin, B., Gibson, M., O'Rear, J., & Harmon, P. (May–June, 1999). A national survey of herbal preparation use by nurse-midwives for labor stimulation: review of the literature and recommendations for practice. *Journal of Nurse Midwifery, 44*(3), 183–188, 205–216.

McGuffin, M., Hobbs, C., Upton, R., & Goldberg, A. (1997). *Botanical safety handbook.* Boca Raton, FL: CRC Press.

McKenna, D. J., Jones, Humphrey, S., & Hughes, K. Black cohosh: Efficacy, safety, and use in clinical and preclinical applications. *Alternative Therapies Health and Medicine, 7*(3), 93–100.

Murray, M. (1995). *The Healing Power of Herbs.* Roseville, CA: Prima Publishing.

Ramsey, L., et al. (February 2000). Efficacy, safety, reliability: Common concerns about herbal products. *Advance for Nurse Practitioners,* 31–33, 86.

Stoll, W. (1987). Phytotherapy influences atrophic vaginal epithelium. *Therapeutikon, 1,* 23. Cited in S. Lieberman (1998). A review of the effectiveness of *Cimicifuga racemosa* (black cohosh) for the symptoms of menopause. *Journal of Women's Health, 7*(5):525–529.

Werbach, M., & Murray, M. (1994). *Botanical influences on illness: A source book of clinical research.* CA: Third Line Press.

NOTES

NOTES

BLACK COHOSH
(Cimicifuga racemosa)

Historical Uses

In China, black cohosh root has been used for centuries for menopausal symptoms and women's health. Native Americans and Eclectic physicians used black cohosh for rheumatism, menstrual difficulties, and sore throats. Don't confuse black cohosh with blue cohosh.

Growth

Black cohosh is a member of the buttercup family. It grows in sunny areas in temperate zones. An at-risk endangered herb, black cohosh can be grown in herb gardens and the roots harvested after 2 years.

Part Used

• Root

Medical Uses

Studies show that black cohosh is helpful in relieving menopausal symptoms, including mood swings, hot flashes, profuse sweating, and sleep disturbances. It has been the largest-selling herbal dietary supplement for menopause in the United States.

Dosage

Tincture or tablets: 40 drops of standardized tincture or one 40-mg tablet twice a day, standardized to 4 mg of triterpenes (a chemical component) for up to 6 months.

Remifemin: The German product Remifemin is also available in the United States; the suggested dosage is 1 tablet twice a day.

Tea: To use herb as a decoction, bring 1 teaspoon of black cohosh root to a boil in 8 ounces of water, simmer about 15 minutes, strain, and drink up to 3 times a day

Warnings

• This herb may cause occasional gastrointestinal discomfort.
• Don't use black cohosh if you're pregnant because this herb stimulates the uterus.
• Don't use black cohosh if you're breast-feeding.
• This herb isn't recommended for children.

- The use of black cohosh with hormone therapy hasn't been studied; check with your primary health-care practitioner before taking this combination.

BROMELAIN
(Ananas comosus)

Historical Uses

In folk medicine, bromelian fruit latex was used to treat wounds, burns, and cancer. It was also used as an aid to digestion (Taussig & Batkin, 1988).

Growth

Commercial bromelain is derived from pineapple stems. The major producers of bromelain are Japan, Taiwan, and Hawaii (Leung, 1980).

Part Used

• Pineapple plant stem

Major Chemical Compounds

• Sulfur-containing proteolytic enzymes (Werbach & Murray, 1994)
• Glycoproteins
• Vitamins that contain enzymes

Clinical Uses

This herb has been used to help resolve hematoma after oral surgery and episiotomy. It has also been used as an anti-inflammatory, an antibiotic, a treatment for cancer and sports injuries, an aid to wound healing (Murray, 1995; *Natural Medicines*, 2000; Werbach & Murray, 1994), and a treatment for mild ulcerative colitis (Kane & Goldberg, 2000). It is approved by the German Commission E for "acute post-op and post-traumatic conditions of swelling, especially of the nasal and paranasal sinuses" (Blumenthal et al., 2000).

Mechanism of Action

This proteolytic enzyme has fibrinolytic effects that decrease kininogen and bradykinin in serum by up to 60 percent. It acts at the level of thromboxane synthetase, decreasing levels of proinflammatory prostaglandins and perhaps re-establishing the balance between proinflammatory and anti-inflammatory prostaglandins (Murray, 1995).

Dosage

The recomended dosage is 80 to 320 mg two or three times daily on an empty stomach for 8 to 10 days.

Side Effects

Bromelain may increase bleeding time.

Contraindications

• Bromelain should not be used by persons with allergy to pineapple.

Herb-Drug Interactions

Bromelain may increase bleeding when taken with anticoagulants. It may increase plasma and urine levels of tetracycline (Blumenthal et al., 1998). It also enhances the effect of penicillin, chloramphenicol, erythromycin, and novobiocin (Neurauer, 1961) and can improve the efficacy of 5-fluorouracil and vincristine (Taussig & Batkin, 1988).

Pregnancy and Breast-Feeding

No restrictions are known (Blumenthal et al., 2000).

SUMMARY OF STUDIES

Kane & Goldberg (2000). Two case studies on the successful use of bromelain in the treatment of mild ulcerative colitis.

Smyth et al. (1967). Biochemical studies on the resolution of inflammation in animals who were treated with bromelain.

REFERENCES

Blumenthal, M. (2000). Interactions between herbs and conventional drugs: Introductory considerations. *HerbalGram, 49*, 52–63.

Blumenthal, M., Busse, W., Goldberg, A., Gruenwald, J., Hall, T., Riggins, C., & Rister, R. (Eds.). (1998). *The complete German Commission E monographs: Therapeutic guide to herbal medicines*. (S. Klein & R. Rister, Trans.). Austin, TX: American Botanical Council; Newton, MA: Integrative Medicine Communications.

Blumenthal, M., Goldberg, A., & Brinckmann, J. (Eds.). (2000). *Herbal medicine expanded Commission E monographs*. Austin, TX: American Botanical Council; Newton, MA: Integrative Medicine Communications.

Kane, S., & Goldberg, M. (2000) Use of bromelain in the treatment of mild ulcerative colitis. *Annals of Internal Medicine, 132*(8), 680.

Leung, A. (1980). *Encyclopedia of common natural ingredients used in foods, drugs and cosmetics* (pp. 74–76). New York: John Wiley & Sons.

Neurauer, R. (1961). A plant protease for potentiation of and possible replacement of antibiotics. *Experimental Medicine and Surgery, 19*, 143–160. Cited in HerbalGram, 49, 58.

Smyth, R., Moss, J., Brennan, R., Harris, J., & Martin, G. (1967). Biochemical studies on the resolution of experimental inflammations in animals treated with bromelain. *Exp Med Surg, 25,* 229–235.

Taussig, S., & Batkin, S. (1988). Bromelain, the enzyme complex of pineapple and its clinical application. An update. *Journal of Ethnopharmacology, 22,* 191–203.

NOTES

NOTES

BROMELAIN
(Ananas comosus)

Historical Uses

In folk medicine, bromelain fruit latex was used to treat wounds, burns, and cancer. It was also used as an aid to digestion.

Growth

Commercial bromelain is derived from pineapple stems. The major producers of bromelain are Japan, Taiwan, and Hawaii.

Part Used

• Pineapple plant stem

Medical Uses

Bromelain is used to decrease swelling after oral surgery and episiotomy. It is also used as an anti-inflammatory, an antibiotic, a treatment for cancer and sports injuries, an aid to wound healing, and a treatment for mild ulcerative colitis.

Dosage

The recommended dosage is 80 to 320 mg two or three times a day on an empty stomach for 8 to 10 days.

Warnings

• Bromelain may increase your risk of bleeding, especially if you take a blood thinner.
• Don't use bromelain if you're allergic to pineapples.
• Discuss the use of this herb with your health-care practitioner if you are taking tetracycline, penicillin, chloramphenicol, erythromycin, novobiocin, or 5-fluorouracil and vincristine.
• No restrictions are known for pregnant or breast-feeding women.

CAYENNE PEPPER

(Capsicum annuum)

Historical Uses

Cayenne pepper (capsaicin) was first used medicinally by a physician during Columbus's voyage (Bown, 1995).

Growth

This mildly pungent plant may be either annual or biennial. Its dark green fruits turn red when ripe.

Part Used

• Fruit

Major Chemical Compounds

• Capsaicinoids, including capsaicin
• Vitamins A, C, and E

Clinical Uses

Cayenne pepper is used for neuralgias and herpes zoster (Zhang & Li Wan Po, 1994) and is effective in the treatment of peptic ulcer (Zhang & Li Wan Po, 1994; Borrelli & Izzo, 2000). It is approved by the German Commission E for "painful muscle spasms of the shoulder, arm, and spine in adults and children" (Blumenthal et al., 2000). It has been shown to be useful for swallowing difficulty in acute tonsillitis (Rau, 2000).

Mechanism of Action

Capsaicin draws blood to the gastrointestinal tract for rapid healing. It also stops Substance P in the pain cycle (Tyler, 1993). *Capsicum* species contain antinociceptive substances, which help to relieve chronic pain (Calixto et al., 2000).

Dosage

External use: 1/2 ounce of cayenne powder added to 1 quart of rubbing alcohol for muscle aches; applied as a poultice.

Ointment or cream: Preparations of .02 to .05 percent capsaicinoids in emulsion base applied to affected areas (Blumenthal et al., 2000). Cream may be applied up to four times a day.

Capsules or tablets: 400 mg to 500 mg up to three times a day (Foster, 1998).

Side Effects

Cayenne pepper may cause a burning sensation when used topically. It can also cause gastrointestinal irritation if taken internally in large doses (McGuffin et al., 1997). It may increase bleeding time.

Contraindications

- Do not give this herb internally if patient has gastrointestinal bleeding.
- Do not rub cayenne in or near the eyes.
- Do not use on open skin.

Herb-Drug Interactions

Chili pepper (cayenne pepper) reduced mucosal damage when taken 30 minutes before aspirin (Yeoh et al., 1995).

Pregnancy and Breast-Feeding

No restrictions are known.

 # SUMMARY OF STUDIES

Yeoh et al. (1995). Cayenne pepper protected 18 subjects' gastric mucosa from aspirin irritation when they took it 30 minutes before taking the aspirin.

Zhang & Li Wan Po (1994). This report is a meta-analysis of the benefits of using capsaicin for osteoarthritis, postherpetic neuralgia, diabetic neuropathy, and psoriasis.

Borrelli & Izzo (2000). The use of *capsicum* as an anti-ulcer remedy was studied.

Calixto et al. (2000). The use of *capsicum* species as naturally occurring antinociceptive substances from plants was studied.

Rau, E (2000). A mixture of *capsicum* and other herbs in a clinical trial of 48 patients with acute tonsillitis alleviated swallowing difficulty within the first 5 days of treatment in more than half of the patients, with no side effects noted.

REFERENCES

Blumenthal, M., Goldberg, A., & Brinckmann, J. (Eds.). (2000). *Herbal medicine expanded Commission E monographs.* Austin, TX: American Botanical Council; Newton, MA: Integrative Medicine Communications.

Borrelli, F., & Izzo, A. (2000). The plant kingdom as a source of anti-ulcer remedies. *Phytotherapy Research, 14*(8), 581–591.

Bown, D. (1995). *The Herb Society of America encyclopedia of herbs and their uses.* New York: Dorling Kindersley Publishing.

Calixto, J.B., Beirith, A., Ferreira, J., Santos, A. R., Filho, V. C., & Yunes, R. A. (2000). Naturally occurring antinociceptive substances from plants. *Phytotherapy Research, 14*(6), 401–418.

Foster, S. (1998). *101 medicinal herbs.* Loveland, CO: Interweave Press.

McGuffin, M., Hobbs, C., Upton, R., & Goldberg, A. (1997). *Botanical safety handbook* (p. 23). Boca Raton, FL: CRC Press.

Rau, E. (2000). Treatment of acute tonsillities with a fixed-combination herbal preparation. *Advances in Therapy, 17*(4), 197–203.

Tyler, V. (1993). *The honest herbal.* Binghamton, NY: Pharmaceutical Products Press.

Yeoh, K., Kang, Y., Yap, I., Guan, R., Tan, C. C., Wee, A., & Teng, C. H. Chili protects against aspirin-induced gastroduodenal mucosal injury in humans. *Digestive Diseases and Sciences, 40*(3), 580–583.

Zhang, W., & Li Wan Po (1994). The effectiveness of topically applied capsaicin. A meta-analysis. *European Journal of Clinical Pharmacology, 46*(6), 517–522.

NOTES

CAYENNE PEPPER
(Capsicum annuum)

Historical Uses

Cayenne pepper was first used medicinally by a physician during Columbus's voyage.

Growth

This mildly pungent plant may be either annual or biennial. Its dark green fruits turn red when ripe.

Part Used

• Fruit

Medical Uses

Cayenne pepper (capsaicin) is used for peptic ulcer disease, neuralgias, and herpes zoster.

Dosage

External use: ¹/₂ ounce cayenne powder to 1 quart of rubbing alcohol for muscle aches, applied as a poultice.

Ointment or cream: Preparations of .02 to .05 percent capsaicinoids in emulsion base applied to affected areas. Cream may be applied up to four times a day.

Capsules or tablets: 400 mg to 500 mg up to three times a day.

Warnings

• Topical use can cause a burning sensation.
• Cayenne pepper may increase your risk of bleeding.
• Don't rub cayenne pepper in or near your eyes.
• If you take aspirin, talk with your health-care practitioner about taking cayenne before taking aspirin. In a clinical study, chili (cayenne) pepper taken 30 minutes before aspirin reduced damage to the lining of the gastrointestinal tract that can result from aspirin.

• Internal use of large doses can cause gastrointestinal irritation.
• Don't use this herb if you have gastrointestinal bleeding.
• Don't use this herb on broken skin.
• No restrictions are noted during pregnancy or breast-feeding.

RECIPES

SORE MUSCLE RUB

For external use only. To ease sore muscles, add ½ ounce of cayenne powder to 1 quart of rubbing alcohol. Or chop a red pepper, add to rubbing alcohol, and let the mixture sit until the alcohol turns red. Then strain out the pepper pieces. Rub either preparation onto your skin to help ease sore muscles. Don't apply it on open wounds or near your eyes. Don't take it internally.

STRESS REDUCERS

If you have gastroesophageal reflux disease or a similar digestive disorder, try these stress-reduction "recipes" to help yourself relax, increase the oxygen flow in your body, and decrease your heart rate.

Belly breathing. While lying or sitting, close your eyes and place both hands on your belly. As you breathe in through your nose, feel your stomach push out into your hands. As you breathe out through your mouth, feel your stomach pull in. Try this three times. Then hold your breath for a few seconds and enjoy this peaceful, restful time.

If you have trouble going to sleep at night, do a few belly breaths with your eyes closed. If thoughts come into your mind, just start counting each breath as you exhale. If you still have trouble going to sleep, play an audiotape of the sounds of gentle waves. Inhale as each wave recedes, and exhale as each wave comes to shore.

Exercise. Get some form of exercise daily, such as a meditative walk. Or try lying face up with your back on a huge exercise ball; relax to help stretch your stomach area. During your exercise time, make sure to get plenty of sunshine and fresh air.

Meditation. Either lie down or sit comfortably in a chair with your feet flat on the floor and your hands in lap. Make sure the room is quiet, the phone is off the hook, and the door is closed. Or go for a quiet walk in the woods and lean up against a tree. Close your eyes. Take a deep breath in through your nose and breathe out through your mouth. As you inhale, feel your stomach push out. As you exhale, feel your stomach pull in. Relax and think of a peaceful image. Or, if you choose, think of a word such as "peace" or "love" and repeat it in your mind. Relax for about 10 minutes. Do this exercise at least once a day.

CHAMOMILE
(Matricaria chamomilla)

Historical Uses

Chamomile is also known as scented mayweed and German chamomile. Many cultures associated chamomile with healing. In the well-known story, Peter Rabbit's mother gave Peter chamomile tea to help relieve his stomachache. Chamomile has been used for stomach discomforts, colic, and teething. It also has been used to promote relaxation.

Growth

Chamomile is an annual herb of the aster or composite family. Easy to grow in the garden, chamomile likes acidic soil, lots of sun, and good drainage. It grows to about 3 feet tall and has small daisylike flowers. The leaves are very fragile and feathery.

Part Used

- Flower heads

Major Chemical Compounds

- Bisabolol
- Chamazulene
- Flavonoids: quercetin and apigenin
- Volatile oils (Tyler, 1993)

Clinical Uses

Chamomile is used internally for the gastrointestinal tract and nervous system. It is also used internally for its anti-inflammatory, anti-allergic, and antispasmodic effects. It is used externally for skin and mucous membrane inflammation and hemorrhoids (*Natural Medicines*, 2000).

Chamomile is approved by the German Commission E for "internal use of gastrointestinal spasms and inflammation and externally for skin and inflammation of the mucous membranes" (Blumenthal et al., 2000). It is approved by the World Health Organization for "internal digestive complaints and external skin inflammations and hemorrhoids" (Blumenthal et al., 2000).

Chamomile is used for babies to help with sleep, colic, and teething (Scott, 1990).

Mechanism of Action

Bisabolol causes rapid healing and soothing of the gastrointestinal tract (Tyler, 1994). Spasmolytic effects are thought to inhibit leukotriene synthesis. Polysaccharides activate macrophages and B lymphocytes for wound healing. Proazulenes contained in the flower are anti-allergenic. Apigenin causes the relaxing effect. Many active constituents of chamomile, rather than one major chemical compound, are responsible for its actions. (Tyler, 1993).

Dosage

The Food and Drug Administration lists chamomile as an herb that is generally recognized as safe. Use Young's or Clark's rule (see Chap. 4) to calculate dosages for children.

Extracts: Standardized to 1.2 percent apigenin.

Capsules: 350 mg to 500 mg up to four times a day.

Tea: By infusion for adults, 1 cup three times daily and at bedtime. Infuse 3 grams of chamomile in 150 mL of water, steep for 5 minutes, then strain. The tea must be covered while steeping to prevent volatile oils from escaping. The tea may also be used as a mouthwash for mouth sores or inflammation of the mucous membranes (Blumenthal et al., 2000).

Tincture: (1:5) (g/mL) taken as 15 mL three or four times a day.

Herbal bath: For dry skin and relaxation, mix 1 quart of nonfat milk powder with 1/2 cup of ground oatmeal. Add 1/4 cup of crushed chamomile flowers. Mix with warm bath water or put into cotton bath sack and float in the bath water. Tell patient to soak for about 15 minutes, rinse, and dry.

Side Effects

Chamomile pollen may cause hypersensitivity reactions.

Contraindications

Chamomile is contraindicated in patients who are allergic to chrysanthemums, ragweed, asters, goldenrod, marigold, daisies, or other herbs.

Herb-Drug Interactions

None are known.

Pregnancy and Breast-Feeding

No restrictions are known (Blumenthal et al., 2000).

Pediatric Patients

Chamomile is safe for use in colic (Weizman et al., 1993), sleep disorders, and teething (Scott, 1990).

SUMMARY OF STUDIES

Weizman et al. (1993). This randomized, double-blind, placebo-controlled study included 69 infants with colic who drank a mixture of chamomile and other herbs in the form of herbal tea. Results: 57 percent had a reduction of colic symptoms. Dosages were up to 150 mL up to 3 times a day. No side effects were observed.

REFERENCES

Blumenthal, M., Goldberg, A., & Brinckmann, J. (Eds.). (2000). *Herbal medicine expanded Commission E monographs.* Austin, TX: American Botanical Council; Newton, MA: Integrative Medicine Communications.

Natural Medicines Comprehensive Database. (2000). *Pharmacist's Letter and Prescriber's Letter.* Therapeutic Research Faculty.

Scott, J.(1990). *Natural medicine for children.* London: Gaia.

Tyler, V. (1994). *Herbs of choice.* Binghamton, NY: Pharmaceutical Products Press.

Tyler, V. (1993). *The honest herbal.* Binghamton, NY: Pharmaceutical Products Press.

Weizman, Z., Alkrinawi, S., Goldfarb, D., & Bitran, C. (1993). Efficacy of herbal tea preparation in infantile colic. *The Journal of Pediatrics, 122,* 650–652.

NOTES

NOTES

CHAMOMILE
(Matricaria chamomilla)

Historical Uses

Chamomile is also known as scented mayweed and German chamomile. Many cultures associated chamomile with healing. In the well-known story, Peter Rabbit's mother gave Peter chamomile tea to help relieve his stomachache. Chamomile has been used for stomach discomforts, colic, and teething. It also has been used to promote relaxation.

Growth

Chamomile is an annual herb of the aster or composite family. Easy to grow in the garden, chamomile likes acidic soil, lots of sun, and good drainage. It grows to about 3 feet tall and has small daisylike flowers. The leaves are very fragile and feathery.

Part Used

• Flower heads

Medical Uses

This herb is used internally for the gastrointestinal tract and nervous system and for its anti-inflammatory, anti-allergic, and antispasmodic effects. It is used externally for skin and mucous membrane inflammation and hemorrhoids. Chamomile is used for babies to help with sleep, colic, and teething.

Dosage

Ask your health-care practitioner about dosages for children.

Extracts: Standardized to 1.2 percent apigenin.

Capsules: 350 mg to 500 mg up to four times a day.

Tea: By infusion for adults, 1 cup three times daily and at bedtime. Infuse 3 grams of chamomile in 150 mL of water, steep for 5 minutes, and then strain. The tea must be covered while steeping to prevent volatile oils from escaping. The tea may also be used as a mouthwash for mouth sores or inflammation of the mucous membranes.

Tincture: (1:5) (g/mL), taken as 15 mL three or four times a day.

Herbal bath: For dry skin and relaxation, mix 1 quart of nonfat milk powder with ½ cup of ground oatmeal. Add ¼ cup of crushed chamomile flowers. Mix with warm bath water or put into cotton bath sack and float in the bath water. Soak for about 15 minutes, rinse, and dry.

Warnings

- Don't use this herb if you're hypersensitive (allergic) to the pollen.
- Don't use this herb if you're allergic to chrysanthemums, ragweed, asters, goldenrod, marigold, daisies, or other herbs.
- No herb-drug interactions are known.
- This herb is safe for use during pregnancy and breast-feeding if consumed in appropriate amounts.
- Chamomile is safe for use in colic, sleep disorders, and teething in children.

RECIPES

RELAXING FOOT BATH

Add ¼ cup of chamomile flowers to 2 quarts of warm water, strain the flowers, and soak your feet for about 15 minutes. Light candles, play soothing music, and relax.

STRESS REDUCERS

If you have a digestive or nervous system disorder, try these stress-reduction "recipes" to help yourself relax, increase the oxygen flow in your body, and decrease your heart rate.

Belly Breathing. While lying or sitting, close your eyes and place both hands on your belly. As you breathe in through your nose, feel your stomach push out into your hands. As you breathe out through your mouth, feel your stomach pull in. Try this three times. Then hold your breath for a few seconds and enjoy this peaceful, restful time.

If you have trouble going to sleep at night, do a few belly breaths with your eyes closed. If thoughts come into your mind, just start counting each breath as you exhale. If you still have trouble going to sleep, play an audiotape of the sounds of gentle waves. Inhale as each wave recedes and exhale as each wave comes to shore.

Exercise. Get some form of exercise daily, such as a meditative walk. Or try lying face up with your back on a huge exercise ball; relax to help stretch your stomach area. During your exercise time, make sure to get plenty of sunshine and fresh air.

Meditation. Either lie down or sit comfortably in a chair with your feet flat on the floor and your hands in your lap. Make sure the room is quiet, the phone is off the hook, and the door is closed. Or go for a quiet walk in the woods and lean against a tree. Close your eyes. Take a deep breath in through your nose and breathe out through your mouth. As you inhale, feel your stomach push out. As you exhale, feel your stomach pull in. Relax, and think of a peaceful image. Or, if you choose, think of a word such as "peace" or "love" and repeat it in your mind. Relax for about 10 minutes. Do this exercise at least once a day.

CHASTE TREE BERRY
(Vitex agnus-castus)

Historical Uses

Long associated with chastity and virtue, this herb is also known as "monk's pepper" and chasteberry. In folklore, chaste tree berry was used for menstrual problems and to increase milk flow.

Growth

Chaste trees grow in the southern United States. The berries look and smell like peppercorns.

Part Used

• Fruit

Major Active Compounds

• Flavonoids
• Agnuside

Clinical Uses

Chaste tree berry is used for premenstrual syndrome (Klepser & Nisly, 1999; Lauritzen et al., 1997; Hardy, 2000; Schellenberg, 2001) and for menopausal and menstrual symptoms (Liu et al., 2001). It is approved by the German Commission E for "menstrual irregularities, PMS, and mastodynia" (breast tenderness) (Blumenthal et al., 2000).

Mechanism of Action

Chaste tree berries work to balance progesterone and estrogen and decrease prolactin levels (McCaleb et al., 2000). They have shown significant competitive binding to estrogen receptors alpha and beta and have stimulated a progesterone receptor (Liu et al., 2001).

Dosage

Tea: Pour 1 cup of boiling water onto 1 teaspoon (0.5 to 1 g) of ripe berries and let sit for 10 to 15 minutes. The tea may be taken up to three times a day.

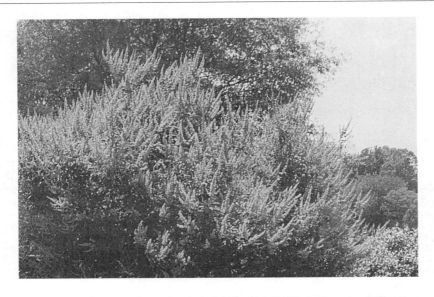

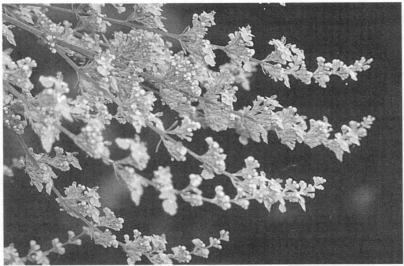

Standardized vitex extract: 40 drops once a day. Standardized to 0.6 percent agnuside (McCaleb et al., 2000).

Tincture: May be taken at 40 drops three times a day. Studies used 20 to 40 mg of dried berry extract standardized to contain 0.5 percent agnuside. Chaste tree berry may be taken for 6 months to a year (McCaleb et al., 2000).

Capsules: Because each brand differs in amount, capsules should be taken as directed.

Side Effects

Side effects may include itching, gastrointestinal complaints, and headache.

Contraindications

• This herb is contraindicated during pregnancy and breast-feeding.

Herb-Drug Interactions

In animal studies, chaste tree berry had a dopaminergic effect. Therefore caution is warranted during use with dopamine-receptor antagonists (i.e., haloperidol) (Blumenthal et al., 1998). Caution is also warranted during use with metoclopramide, hormone therapy, or oral contraceptives because the herb may counteract their effects (Blumenthal, 2000).

Pregnancy and Breast-Feeding

Do not use chaste tree berry in pregnant women because it has uterine stimulant properties (Blumenthal, 2000; McGuffin et al., 1997). Also avoid use in breast-feeding women.

Pediatric Patients

This herb is not used in children (McCaleb et al., 2000).

 # SUMMARY OF STUDIES

Loch et al. (2000). This open, uncontrolled study took place over 3 months and included 1634 women with premenstrual syndrome. Results: Patients reported a decrease in the number of symptoms and even cessation of premenstrual complaints, with good tolerability.

Klepser & Nisly (1999). Several studies concluded that women had a significant reduction in premenstrual syndrome symptoms. Efficacy in physician reports exceeded 90 percent, and 57 percent of patients reported improvement in their symptoms.

Lauritzen et al. (1997). A controlled, randomized, double-blind study of 175 women over a 3-month period compared the use of vitex and pyridoxine for premenstrual syndrome. Vitex capsules contained 3.5 to 4.2 mg dried chaste tree berry extract. Product: Agnolyt of Germany, plus one placebo capsule (n=90), or two 100-mg capsules of pyridoxine (n=85). Results: Vitex improved and alleviated symptoms of premenstrual syndrome better than pyridoxine did. Both groups reported mild side effects including headache, gastrointestinal and abdominal complaints, and skin problems.

Schellenberg (2001). A study of 178 women given chaste tree berry or placebo in doses of one tablet daily for three consecutive cycles showed that chaste tree berry was effective and well tolerated for relief of the symptoms of premenstrual tension.

REFERENCES

Blumenthal, M. (2000). Interactions between herbs and conventional drugs: Introductory considerations. *HerbalGram, 49,* 52–63.

Blumenthal, M., Busse, W., Goldberg, A., Gruenwald, J., Hall, T., Riggins, C., & Rister, R. (Eds.). (1998). *The complete German Commission E monographs: Therapeutic guide to herbal medicines.* (S. Klein & R. Rister, Trans.); Austin, TX: American Botanical Council; Newton, MA: Integrative Medicine Communications.

Blumenthal M, Goldberg A, Brinckmann J. (eds.). (2000). *Herbal Medicine Expanded Commission E Monographs,* Austin, TX: American Botanical Council; Newton, MA:: Integrative Medicine Communications (pp. 62–63, 479).

Hardy, M. L. (2000). Herbs of special interest to women. *Journal of the American Pharmaceutical Association, 40*(2), 234–242.

Klepser, T., & Nisly, N. (June 1999). Chaste tree berry for premenstrual syndrome. *Alternative Medicine Alert,* 63–66.

Lauritzen, C., et al. (1997). Treatment of premenstual tension syndrome with *Vitex agnus-castus.* Controlled, double-blind study versus pyrodoxine. *Phytomedicine, 4*(3), 183–189.

Liu, J., Burdette, J. E., Xu, H., Gu, C., van Breemen, R. B., Bhat, K. B., Booth, N, Constantinou, A. I., Pezzuto, J. M., Fong, H. H., Farnsworth, N. R., & Bolton, J. L. (2001). Evaluation of estrogenic activity of plant extracts for the potential treatment of menopausal symptoms. *Journal of Agricultural and Food Chemistry, 49*(5), 2472–2479.

Loch, E.G., Selle, H., & Boblitz, N. (April 2000). Treatment of premenstrual syndrome with a phytopharma-ceutical formulation containing *Vitex agnus castus. Journal of Womens Health Gender-Based Medicine, 9*(3), 315–320.

McCaleb, R., Leigh, E., & Morien, K. (2000). *The encyclopedia of popular herbs.* Roseville, CA: Prima Publishing.

McGuffin, M., Hobbs, C., Upton, R., & Goldberg, A. (1997). *Botanical safety handbook.* Boca Raton, FL: CRC Press.

Schellenberg, R. (2001). Treatment for the premenstrual syndrome with *Agnus castus* fruit extract: Prospective, randomized, placebo controlled study. *British Medical Journal, 322*(7279), 134–137.

NOTES

CHASTE TREE BERRY
(Vitex agnus-castus)

Historical Uses

Long associated with chastity and virtue, this herb is also known as "monk's pepper" and chasteberry. In folklore, chaste tree berry was used for menstrual problems and to increase milk flow.

Growth

Chaste trees grow in the southern United States. The berries look and smell like peppercorns.

Part Used

• Fruit

Medical Uses

Chaste tree berries are used for premenstrual syndrome and for menopausal and menstrual symptoms.

Dosage

Tea: Pour 1 cup of boiling water onto 1 teaspoon (0.5 to 1 g) of ripe berries and let sit for 10 to 15 minutes. Tea may be taken up to three times daily.

Standardized vitex extract: 40 drops once daily. Standardized to 0.6 percent agnuside.

Tincture: May be taken at 40 drops three times daily. Studies used 20 to 40 mg of dried berry extract standardized to contain 0.5 percent agnuside. Chaste tree berry may be taken for 6 months to a year.

Capsules: Because each brand differs in amount, capsules should be taken as directed.

Warnings

• Side effects may include itching, gastrointestinal complaints, and headache.
• Discuss use of this herb with your health-care practitioner if you take any of the following medications: haloperidol, metoclopramide, hormone therapy, or oral contraceptives.
• Don't use this herb during pregnancy or breast-feeding.
• This herb is not recommended for children.

COMFREY
(Symphytum officinale)

Historical Uses

In folklore, comfrey was used for healing gastric ulcers and reducing the inflammation around fractures. It is also known as knitbone.

Growth

Comfrey is a perennial plant that grows to about 2 to 4 feet high. It has huge, broad, hairy leaves and a small, bell-shaped flower.

Parts Used

- Leaves
- Root

Major Chemical Compounds

- Allantoin
- Pyrrolizidine alkaloids (more in the roots)
- Mucilage
- Tannins

Clinical Uses

Comfrey is used externally for superficial wounds, sore breasts, and hemorrhoids.

Mechanism of Action

Allantoin promotes cell proliferation (Tyler, 1993; Bown, 1995), reduces inflammation, and controls bleeding. Its astringent properties help to heal hemorrhoids (Bown, 1995). Comfrey is unsafe when used internally (Klepser & Klepser, 1999; Winship KA, 1991; Ridker & McDermott, 1989).

Dosage

EXTERNAL USE ONLY

Comfrey may be used externally up to three times daily. It may be applied to the skin in a compress, poultice, or ointment. Do not use for more than 10 days, and do not exceed 100 µg of pyrrolizidine alkaloids each day (*Natural Medicines,* 2000).

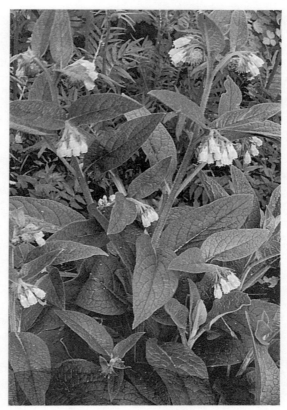

Side Effects

Comfrey may cause veno-occlusive disease (Stickel & Seitz, 2000) and hepatotoxicity and may have carcinogenic effects when taken internally.

Contraindications

- Alkaloids cause liver damage and tumors in cows and laboratory animals when used internally.
- Do not apply comfrey to deep wounds.
- Do not apply comfrey to broken or damaged skin (McGuffin, 2000).

Herb-Drug Interactions

None are known.

Pregnancy and Breast-Feeding

Avoid external use during pregnancy and breast-feeding (*Natural Medicine* 2000; McGuffin et al., 1997).

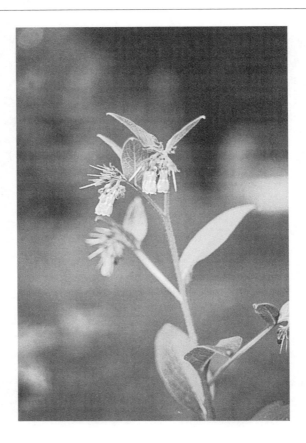

 # SUMMARY OF STUDIES

No recent clinical studies in humans are available.

REFERENCES

Bown, D. (1995). *The Herb Society of America encyclopedia of herbs and their uses.* New York: Dorling Kindersley Publishing.

Klepser, T. B., & Klepser, M. E. (1999). Unsafe and potentially safe herbal therapies. *American Journal of Health-System Pharmacology, 56*(2), 125–138.

McGuffin, M. (2000). Self regulatory initiatives by the herbal industry. *HerbalGram, 48*, 42–43.

McGuffin, M., Hobbs, C., Upton, R., & Goldberg, A. (1997). *Botanical safety handbook.* Boca Raton, FL: CRC Press.

Natural Medicines Comprehensive Database. (2000). *Pharmacist's Letter and Prescriber's Letter.* Therapeutic Research Faculty.

Ridker, P. M., & McDermott, W. V. (1989). Comfrey herb tea and hepatic veno-occlusive disease. *The Lancet, 1*(8639), 657–658.

Stickel, F., & Seitz, H. K. The efficacy and safety of comfrey. *Public Health Nutrition, 3*(4A), 501–508.

Tyler, V. (1993). *The honest herbal*. Binghamton, NY: Pharmaceutical Products Press.

Winship, K. A. (1991). Toxicity of comfrey. *Adverse Drug Reactions Toxicology Review, 10*(1), 47–59.

NOTES

NOTES

COMFREY
(Symphytum officinale)

Historical Uses

In folklore, comfrey was used for healing gastric ulcers and reducing the inflammation around fractures. It was also known as knitbone.

Growth

Comfrey is a perennial plant that grows to about 2 to 4 feet high. It has huge, broad, hairy leaves and a small, bell-shaped flower.

Parts Used

• Leaves
• Root

Medical Uses

Comfrey is used externally for superficial wounds, sore breasts, and hemorrhoids.

Dosage

EXTERNAL USE ONLY

Comfrey may be used externally up to 3 times daily. It may be applied to the skin in a compress, poultice, or ointment. Don't use it for more than 10 days, and don't exceed 100 μg of pyrrolizidine alkaloids each day.

Warnings

• Comfrey may block veins, damage the liver, and cause cancer if taken orally.
• Don't apply comfrey to deep wounds.
• Don't apply comfrey to broken or damaged skin.
• No herb-drug interactions are known.
• Pregnant and breast-feeding women should avoid use of comfrey.

RECIPES

COMFREY OINTMENT

To help heal wounds, you may make an ointment by adding 3 ounces of chopped comfrey to about 6 or 7 ounces of petroleum or nonpetroleum jelly. Simmer (don't boil) the mixture. Then remove from heat, strain the herb, and place the remaining ointment in small jars. Label and date the jars.

CRANBERRY
(Vaccinium macrocarpon)

Historical Uses

Native Americans and Europeans who settled in the United States used cranberries for food and medicinal purposes. Around 1923, scientists discovered that people who consumed cranberries had more acidic urine than those who did not.

Growth

The cranberry is related to the blueberry and bilberry. Cranberries prefer bogs, cool weather, and acidic soils.

Part Used

- Fruit (red berries)

Major Chemical Compounds

- Proanthocyanidins
- Flavonoids
- Fructose
- Vitamin C

Clinical Uses

Cranberries are used to prevent urinary tract infections (UTIs) and are useful in treating mild UTIs (Kontiokari et al., 2001).

Mechanism of Action

Cranberry prevents the adherence of bacteria to the walls of the urinary tract (Zafrifi et al., 1989; Howell et al., 1998; Foo et al., 2000) because the fructose compound inhibits adhesion of *Escherichia coli* (Zafrifi et al., 1989) and proanthocyanidins inhibit adhesion of *E. coli* to uroepithelial cells (Howell et al., 1998).

Dosage

Capsules: 300 to 400 mg twice a day of standardized, concentrated cranberry extract capsules.

Berries or juice: The daily amount needed is 1½ ounces of fresh or frozen cranberries or 3 ounces of cranberry juice. For prevention, use one daily serving of cranberries or cranberry juice cocktail. For treatment, 4 to 10 servings, or up to 32 ounces per day, may be needed.

Side Effects

None are known.

Contraindications

None are known.

Herb-Drug Interactions

None are known.

Pregnancy and Breast-Feeding

Cranberries are safe if used as recommended.

SUMMARY OF STUDIES

Avorn et al. (1994) In this 6-month, double-blind, placebo-controlled study, 153 women drank 300 mL of cranberry juice cocktail or a synthetic placebo drink with a similar flavor but no cranberry content each day. Results: Regular intake of cranberry juice cocktail significantly reduced the frequency of bacteriuria and pyuria in elderly women.

Kontiokari et al. (2001). This was an open, randomized 12-month follow-up of 150 women with UTIs caused by *Escherichia coli.* The women were divided into three groups: the first group drank cranberry-lingonberry juice; the second a lactobacillus GG drink, and the third a placebo drink. The recurrence of UTIs was reduced in the first group only.

REFERENCES

Avorn, J, et al. (1994). Reduction of bacteriuria and pyuria after ingestion of cranberry juice. *Journal of the American Medical Association, 271*(10), 751–754.

Foo, L.Y., Lu, Y., Howell, A. B., & Vorsa, N (2000). The structure of cranberry proanthocyanidins which inhibit adherence of uropathogenic P-fimbriated *Escherichia coli* in vitro. *Phytochemistry, 54*(2), 173–81.

East and West, 5(2), 123–145.

Howell, A. B., Vorsa, N., Der Marderosian, A., & Foo Ly. (1998). Inhibition of the adherence of p-fimbriated *Escherichia coli* to uroepithelial-cell surfaces by proanthocyanidin extracts from cranberries. *New England Journal of Medicine, 339*(15), 1085–1086.

Kontiokari, T., Sundqvist, K., Nuutinen, M., Pokka, T., & Uhari, M. (2001). Randomised trial of cranberry-lingonberry juice and lactobacillus GG drink for the prevention of urinary tract infections in women. *British Medical Journal, 322*(7302), 1571.

Zafriri, D., Ofek, I., Adar, R., Pocino, M., & Sharon, N. (1989). Inhibitory activity of cranberry juice on adherence of type 1 and type P fimbriated *Escherichia coli* to eucaryotic cells. *Antimicrobial Agents and Chemotherapy, 33*(1), 92–98.

NOTES

NOTES

CRANBERRY
(Vaccinium macrocarpon)

Historical Uses

Native Americans and Europeans who settled in the United States used cranberries for food and medicinal purposes. Around 1923, scientists discovered that people who consumed cranberries had more acidic urine than those who did not.

Growth

The cranberry is related to the blueberry and bilberry. Cranberries prefer bogs, cool weather, and acidic soils.

Part Used

• Fruit (red berries)

Medical Uses

Cranberries are used to prevent urinary tract infections and to treat mild urinary tract infections.

Dosage

Capsules: 300 to 400 mg twice a day of standardized, concentrated cranberry extract capsules.

Berries or juice: The daily amount needed is 1½ ounces of fresh or frozen cranberries or 3 ounces of cranberry juice cocktail. For prevention, take one daily serving of cranberries or cranberry juice cocktail. For treatment, 4 to 10 servings, or up to 32 ounces per day, may be needed.

Warnings

• None are known.
• Cranberries are safe if used as recommended for pregnant and breast-feeding women.

DANDELION

(Taraxacum officinale)

Historical Uses

Dandelion first appeared in the 10th century in Arabian medicine and has been used as a diuretic, a treatment for anemia, a blood tonic, a mild laxative, and an appetite stimulant. Europeans used dandelion to treat diabetes. It is reported that dandelion is more nutritious than spinach. It may have antiviral properties that help prevent herpes. It also has been used to treat premenstrual syndrome and hepatitis. It is also called lion's tooth and wild endive.

Growth

Dandelions grow in lawns and fields throughout the spring and summer in the northern hemisphere and are usually considered weeds. The plant has "lion-toothed" leaves and a bright yellow upright flower.

Parts Used

- Leaves
- Roots
- All parts are edible

Major Chemical Compounds

- Chicoric acid
- Monocaffeytartaric acid
- Taraxacin (bitter)
- Taraxacerin
- Sesquiterpene lactones
- Phytosterols
- Iron
- Vitamins A, B, and C

One ounce of fresh dandelion leaves contains large amounts of vitamin A and calcium and moderate amounts of vitamin B_1, vitamin C, sodium, potassium, and trace elements. One cup of dandelion greens provides nearly a day's requirement of vitamin A and one-third the daily requirement of vitamin C. Dandelions contain more calcium than broccoli (Wood, 1999).

Clinical Uses

The root is most often used for liver disease and to increase bile flow. Leaves are used primarily for their diuretic effects and for adolescent acne. The leaf is approved by the German Commission E for "loss of appetite and dyspepsia." The root is approved for "bile flow disturbances, stimulation of diuresis, loss of appetite, and dyspepsia" (Blumenthal et al., 2000). The root is also used as a coffee substitute.

Mechanism of Action

Dandelion is helpful in digestion because the root contains sesquiterpene lactones (Blumenthal et al., 2000) and taraxacin (*Natural Medicines,* 2000). Diuretic effects using dandelion extracts have been noted in animal studies. Increases in bile secretion are thought to result from bitter chemical compounds (Murray, 1995). The leaves are high in vitamin A, which is needed for healthy skin.

Dosage

Fresh greens: Pick fresh dandelion greens in the spring, wash them well, and steam them like spinach. Or add fresh dandelion greens to salads. Add the flowers to vinegars or for food decoration.

Tea: As an infusion, dandelion tea may be consumed up to three times a day. Use one tablespoon of herb and root in 150 mL of water, boil for 5 to 10 minutes, strain, and drink (Blumenthal et al., 2000).

Capsules: 500 to 1000 mg of dried herb up to 4 times a day (Ottariano, 1999).

Side Effects

Dandelion may cause mild intestinal discomfort because of its bitterness. It may also have a laxative effect.

Contraindications

- Dandelion is contraindicated if patient has obstruction of the bile ducts, gallbladder empyema, ileus, or gallstones (Blumenthal et al., 2000; McGuffin et al., 1997).
- Do not collect leaves or roots along roadways or where pesticides have been used.

Herb-Drug Interactions

None are known.

Pregnancy and Breast-Feeding

Dandelion is safe when consumed as a food.

SUMMARY OF STUDIES

No recent clinical studies in humans are available.

REFERENCES

Blumenthal, M., Goldberg, A., & Brinckmann, J. (Eds.). (2000). *Herbal medicine expanded Commission E monographs*. Austin, TX: American Botanical Council; Newton, MA: Integrative Medicine Communications.

McGuffin, M., Hobbs, C., Upton, R., & Goldberg, A. (1997). *Botanical safety handbook* (p. 114). Boca Raton, FL: CRC Press.

Murray, M. (1995). *The Healing Power of Herbs*. Roseville, CA: Prima Publishing.

Natural Medicines Comprehensive Database. (2000). *Pharmacist's Letter and Prescriber's Letter*. Therapeutic Research Faculty.

Ottariano, S. (1999). *Medicinal herbal therapy: A pharmacist's viewpoint*. North Hampton, NH: Nicolin Fields Publishing.

Williams, CA, Goldstone, F., & Greenham, J. (1996. Flavonoids, cinnamic acids and coumarins from the different tissues and medicinal preparations of *Taraxacum officinale*. Phytochemistry, *42*(1), 121–127.

Wood, R. (1999). *The new whole foods encyclopedia* (pp. 106–107). New York: Penguin.

NOTES

DANDELION
(Taraxacum officinale)

Historical Uses

Dandelion first appeared in the 10th century in Arabian medicine and has been used as a diuretic, a treatment for anemia, a blood tonic, a mild laxative, and an appetite stimulant. Europeans used dandelion to treat diabetes. It is reported that dandelion is more nutritious than spinach. It may have antiviral properties that help prevent herpes. It also has been used to treat premenstrual syndrome and hepatitis. It is also called lion's tooth and wild endive.

Growth

Dandelions grow in lawns and fields throughout the spring and summer in the northern hemisphere and are usually considered weeds. The plant has "lion-toothed" leaves and a bright yellow upright flower.

Parts Used

- Leaves
- Roots
- All parts are edible

Medical Uses

Dandelion root is used most often for liver disease and to increase bile flow. The root is also used as a coffee substitute. The leaves are used primarily for their diuretic effect and for adolescent acne.

One ounce of fresh dandelion leaves contains large amounts of vitamin A and calcium and moderate amounts of vitamin B_1, vitamin C, sodium, potassium, and trace elements. One cup of dandelion greens provides nearly a day's requirement of vitamin A and one-third the daily requirement of vitamin C. Dandelions contain more calcium than broccoli.

Dosage

Fresh greens: Pick fresh dandelion greens in the spring, wash them well, and steam them like spinach. Or add fresh dandelion greens to salads. Add the flowers to vinegars or use them for food decoration.

Tea: As an infusion, dandelion tea may be consumed up to three times a day. Use 1 tablespoon of herb and root in 150 mL of water, boil for 5 to 10 minutes, strain, and drink.

Capsules: 500 to 1000 mg of dried herb up to 4 times a day.

Warnings

- Because of its bitterness, dandelion may cause mild intestinal discomfort.
- Dandelion may have a laxative effect.
- Don't take dandelion if you have obstruction of the bile duct, gallbladder problems, or gallstones.
- No herb-drug interactions are known.
- Dandelion is safe for pregnant and breast-feeding women when consumed as a food.

ECHINACEA
(E. angustifolia, E. purpurea, and E. pallida)

Historical Uses

Native Americans and Eclectic physicians used echinacea as a natural anti-infective for colds and flu. Native Americans first introduced echinacea to the colonists.

Growth

There are nine species of echinacea. This perennial will grow in most herb gardens in the northeast. The beautiful flower of *E. purpurea*, commonly called "purple cone-flower," may grow up to 6 feet tall. *E. angustifolia* has narrow leaves and is much shorter, at about 2 feet. It has pink flowers. *E. pallida* grows to about 3 feet and is much paler. All three species have been cultivated in the U.S. and Europe. *E. angustifolia* is listed as an at-risk endangered herb.

Parts Used

- Aerial (above-ground) parts
- Whole plant and root

Major Chemical Compounds

- Alkylamides
- Caffeic acid derivatives
- Cichoric acid
- Polysaccharides
- Glycoproteins

Not all active chemical compounds are found in each species of echinacea.

Mechanism of Action

Alkylamides, which cause a tingling sensation on the tongue, produce anti-inflammatory effects by inhibiting cyclooxygenase. They also stimulate the immune system. The roots of *E. angustifolia* are highest in alkylamides. *E. pallida* contains alkylamides only in the aerial parts of the plant and not in the root.

Caffeic acid inhibits the spread of infection. Cichoric acid causes phagocytosis.

Polysaccharides enhance the immune system and exert wound-healing effects. They activate macrophages. Polysaccharides are the major compounds in *E. purpurea*.

Glycoproteins are highest in *E. purpurea*, which causes the highest stimulation of macrophages and contains cichoric acid.

83

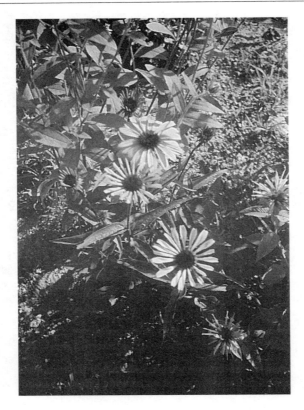

Clinical Uses

Echinacea is used for the common cold, infections, and low immune status. It is also used as adjuvant therapy with antibiotics and chemotherapy and acts as an anti-inflammatory. Recent studies suggest that echinacea appears to work more effectively when taken at the first sign of a cold than when used as a daily preventative (Hoheisel et al., 1997; Lindenmuth, 2000). Echinacea is approved by the German Commission E and the World Health Organization for "supportive therapy of colds, flu, respiratory and urinary infections" (Blumenthal et al., 2000). It also may help in radiation exposure (Foster, 2000). The University of Arizona is currently investigating the use of echinacea in the prevention of recurrent otitis media (Mark et al., 2001).

Dosage

Controversy exists over how echinacea should be standardized; the United States standardizes to a single chemical compound rather than the entire extract, which is more effective (Foster, 2000).

For acute infection: 20 drops of standardized tincture or 1 capsule every 2 hours at the start of a cold for up to 48 hours (Ottariano, 1999). The tincture may be added to a small amount of warm water or juice. After 48 hours, take 30 drops of tincture or

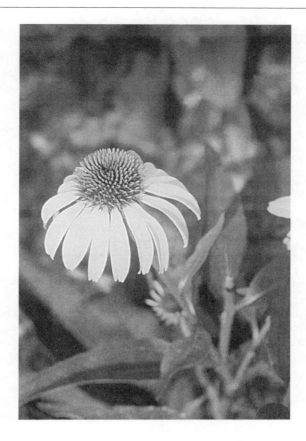

one 300-mg dose of a dry standardized extract three times daily. Chichon (2000) recommends using echinacea as an antibiotic for a maximum of 2 weeks.

For prevention of infections (studies are controversial): 10 to 25 drops daily or 1 to 2 capsules or tablets daily (Hobbs, 1994). During long-term use, it is recommended that the patient spend 1 week without echinacea after every 8 weeks of taking it (Hobbs, 1994).

Side Effects

One case of an anaphylactic reaction has been reported in which the patient had an allergy to ragweed (Mullins, 1998).

Contraindications

- Echinacea should not be used for autoimmune disorders, diabetes mellitus, multiple sclerosis, lupus, AIDS, HIV infection or tuberculosis (Blumenthal et al., 2000).
- Acute toxicity has been noted at dosages over 3 mg/kg.
- Echinacea was adulterated before 1988.

Herb-Drug Interactions

Taking echinacea for more than 8 weeks along with anabolic steroids, methotrexate, amiodarone, or ketoconazole increases the risk of hepatotoxicity. It may have antagonistic effects with immunosuppressants, such as corticosteroids and cyclosporin (Miller, 1998).

Pregnancy and Breast-Feeding

Echinacea is safe with oral use (Parnham, 1996).

Pediatric patients

The children's dose can be calculated using Young's or Clark's rule.

SUMMARY OF STUDIES

Echinacea is well researched, with over 350 studies. All German studies have been done with the expressed juice of *E. purpurea*.

Braunig et al. (1992). In this double-blind, placebo-controlled study of 180 volunteers using an alcohol extract of *E. purpurea* root, echinacea decreased the symptoms and duration of the flu. At 900 mg/day, patients showed a statistically significant improvement in symptoms within 3 to 4 days compared to placebo and to an echinacea dose of 450 mg.

Brinkeborn et al. (1998). In this study, 199 patients took echinacea extract or placebo at the first sign of a cold. Physicians found that echinacea extract was effective in 68 percent of cases, and 78 percent of patients reported that they found it effective. *E. purpurea* aerial parts and root were used and taken in doses of 2 tabs t.i.d. over 8 days. The tablets contained a dosage of extract equal to about 240 mg of echinacea per day. Both patients and physicians agreed that Echinaforce and Bioforce reduced cold symptoms better than placebo.

Hoheisel et al. (1997). In this randomized, double-blind, placebo-controlled clinical trial, 120 patients ingested 20 drops of echinacea every 2 hours for the first day after cold symptoms began and then t.i.d. for up to 10 days. Patients reported that only 40 percent of those who took the echinacea progressed to a cold compared to 60 percent in the placebo group. Patients who took the echinacea had colds that lasted 4 days compared to 8 days in the placebo group.

Shoneberger (1992). In this double-blind, placebo-controlled study, 108 volunteers with chronic upper respiratory infections took 2 to 4 mL/day of *E. purpurea* fresh juice extract. The treatment group had milder symptoms, briefer infections, and a longer period between infections.

Tubaro et al. (1987). Echinacea polysaccharides appear to be slightly inferior in potency to indomethacin. The anti-inflammatory action results from polysaccharides.

Baetgen (1988). This study looked at the treatment of acute bronchitis in children using three groups: one group (n=468) took echinacea juice; one group (n=330) took echinacea and chemotherapeutics; and one group (n=482) took chemotherapeutics alone. Results: After 5 days, 45 percent of the group who took only echinacea experienced a cure. After 10 days, there was no difference between the three groups. Chemotherapeutics did not help viral infections. Tetracycline and chloramphenicol prevented healing.

Stimpel et al. (1984). Polysaccharides of *E. purpurea* were shown to strongly activate macrophages without toxic effects. These results have relevance for tumors and infectious systems.

Currier & Miller (2001). Daily doses of *E. purpurea* in vivo to leukemic mice demonstrated positive effects.

Lindenmuth (2000). In a randomized controlled trial, 95 subjects were given Echinacea Plus tea at the onset of cold and flu symptoms. Results showed that the tea was effective in relieving the symptoms of cold and flu in less time than placebo.

REFERENCES

Baetgen, D. (1988). Treatment of acute bronchitis in children using Echinacin. *Pediatrie, 1,* 66.

Blumenthal, M., Busse, W., Goldberg, A., Gruenwald, J., Hall, T., Riggins, C., & Rister, R. (Eds.). (1998). *The complete German Commission E monographs: Therapeutic guide to herbal medicines* (pp. 88–101, 479). (S. Klein & R. Rister, Trans.). Austin, TX: American Botanical Council; Newton, MA: Integrative Medicine Communications.

Brauning et al. (1992). (S. Coble & C. Hobbs, Trans.). *Echinacea purpurea* radix for strengthening the immune response in flu-like infections. *Zefur Phytotherapie, 13,* 7–13.

Brinkeborn, R., Shah, D., Geissbuhler, S., & Degening, F. H. (1998). Echinaforce in the treatment of acute colds. *Schweiz Zeitschrift GansheitsMedzin, 10,* 26–29.

Chichon, P. (August 2000). Herbs and the common cold. *Advance for Nurse Practitioners,* 31–32.

Currier, N. L., & Miller, S. C. (2001). *Echinacea purpurea* and melatonin augment natural-killer cells in leukemic mice and prolong life span. *Journal of Alternative and Complementary Medicine, 7*(3), 241–251.

Foster, S. (January/February 2000). The latest on echinacea. *Herbs for Health,* 8–9.

Hobbs, C. (1994). Echinacea: A literature review. *HerbalGram,* 30.

Hoheisel, O., Sandberg, M., Bertram, S., Bulitta, M., & Schafer, M: (1997). Echinagard treatment shortens the course of the common cold: A double-blind, placebo-controlled clinical trial. *European Journal of Clinical Research, 9,* 261–268.

Lindenmuth, G. F., & Lindenmuth, E. B. (2000). The efficacy of echinacea compound herbal tea preparation on the severity and duration of upper respiratory and flu symptoms: A randomized, double-blind placebo-controlled study. *Journal of Alternative and Complementary Medicine, 6*(4), 327–334.

Mark, J. D., Grant, K. L., & Barton, L. L. (2001). The use of dietary supplements in pediatrics: A study of echinacea. *Clinical Pediatrics, 40*(5):265–269.

Miller, L. (1998). Herbal medicinals: Selected clinical considerations focusing on known or potential drug-herb interactions. *Archives of Internal Medicine, 158,* 2200–2211. Cited in Vickers & Zollman (1999). Herbal medicine. *British Medical Journal, 319,* 1050–1053.

Mullins, R. (1998). Echinacea-associated anaphylaxis. *Medical Journal of Australia, 16*(4), 170–171.

Ottariano, S. (1999). *Medicinal herbal therapy: A pharmacist's viewpoint.* North Hampton, NH: Nicolin Fields Publishing.

Parnham, M. (1996). Benefit-risk assessment of the squeezed sap of the purple coneflower (*E. purpurea*) for long-term oral immunostimulation. *Phytomedicine, 3*(1), 95–102.

Schoneberger, D. (1992) (Sigrid & Klein, Trans.). The influence of immune stimulant effects of pressed juice from *Echinacea purpurea* on the course and severity of colds. *Forum Immunologie, 8,* 2–12.

Stimpel, M., Proksch, A., Wagner, H., & Lohmann-Matthes, M. (1984). Macrophage activation and induction of macrophage cytotoxicity by purified polysaccharide fractions from the plant *Echinacea purpurea*. *Infection and Immunity, 46*(3), 845–849.

Tubaro, A., Tragni, E., DelNegro, P., Galli, C., & Loggia. (1987). Anti-inflammatory activity of a polysaccharidic fraction of *Echinacea angustifolia*. *Journal of Pharmacognosy and Pharmacology, 39,* 567–569.

NOTES

ECHINACEA
(E. angustifolia, E. purpurea, and E. pallida)

Historical Uses

Native Americans and the eclectic physicians used echinacea as a natural anti-infective for colds and flu. Native Americans first introduced echinacea to the colonists.

Growth

There are nine species of echinacea. This perennial will grow in most herb gardens in the northeast. The beautiful flower of *E. purpurea*, commonly called purple coneflower, may grow up to 6 feet tall. *E. angustifolia* has narrow leaves and is much shorter, at about 2 feet. It has pink flowers. *E. pallida* grows to about 3 feet and is much paler. All three species have been cultivated in the U.S. and Europe. *E. angustifolia* is listed as an at-risk endangered herb.

Parts Used

- Aerial (above-ground) parts
- Whole plant and root

Medical Uses

Echinacea is used for the common cold, infections, and low immune status. It is given with antibiotics and chemotherapy and acts as an anti-inflammatory. Recent studies suggest that echinacea works more effectively when taken at the first sign of a cold than when used as a daily preventative.

Dosage

For acute infection: 20 drops of standardized tincture or one capsule every 2 hours at the start of a cold for up to 48 hours. The tincture may be added to a small amount of warm water or juice. After 48 hours, take 30 drops of tincture or one 300-mg dose of a dry standardized extract three times daily. Use echinacea as an antibiotic for a maximum of 2 weeks.

For prevention of infections (studies are controversial): 10 to 25 drops daily or 1 to 2 capsules or tablets daily. If you take echinacea for a long time, spend 1 week off this herb after every 8 weeks of taking it.

Ask your health-care practitioner about dosages for children.

Warnings

- Echinacea may cause allergy symptoms in some people.
- Don't take echinacea if you have an autoimmune disorder, diabetes mellitus, multiple sclerosis, lupus, AIDS, HIV infection, or tuberculosis.
- Echinacea may be toxic when taken in large amounts.
- Don't take echinacea with any of these medications: anabolic steroids, methotrexate, amiodarone, ketoconazole, corticosteroids, or cyclosporin. Talk with your health-care practitioner.

EVENING PRIMROSE
(Oenothera biennis)

Historical Uses

In the past, evening primrose has been used to treat female complaints, skin problems, and respiratory difficulties.

Growth

Evening primrose is a biennial North American plant with a beautiful, fragrant yellow flower that opens in the evening. It prefers sun and dry soil. The seeds are pressed into oil.

Part Used

• Seed, pressed into oil

Major Chemical Compound

• Gamma-linolenic acid (GLA)

Clinical Uses

Evening primrose is used for diabetic neuropathy, symptoms of premenstrual syndrome (Hardy, 2000), and benign breast pain. It may be beneficial in rheumatic conditions (Belch & Hill, 2000) and atopic eczema (Horrobin DF, 2000). In a survey of certified nursing midwives who used herbal preparations, 60 percent stated that they used evening primrose oil to stimulate labor (McFarlin et al., 1999).

Mechanism of Action

GLA is an essential fatty acid. These acids are essential for keeping cells healthy and for preventing cardiovascular disease, depression, infections, sterility, cancer, and dry hair and skin. Anti-inflammatory properties may be a result of mediation by prostaglandin E_1 (Darlington & Stone, 2001).Evening primrose oil also helps to counter neuropathy by enhancing peripheral blood flow (Guthrie, 2000).

Dosage

Evening primrose oil is standardized to contain 7 to 10 percent GLA (McCaleb et al., 2000).

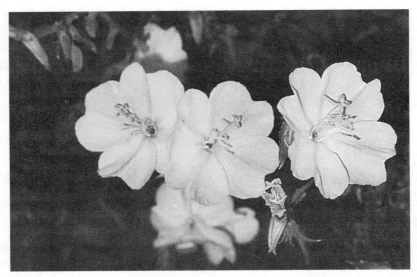

Capsules: 1 to 2 capsules three times daily for premenstrual syndrome, 8 to 12 capsules daily (containing 320–480 mg of total GLA) for diabetic neuropathy, and 6 capsules daily for eczema (McCaleb et al., 2000). Take with meals. It may be several months before an effect is evident.

Side Effects

Evening primrose may cause minor stomach upset, nausea, or headache at high doses (McCaleb et al., 2000).

Contraindications

• None are known.

Herb-Drug Interactions

Evening primrose should not be taken with phenothiazines (Kuhn, 1999; McCaleb et al., 2000). It may decrease the seizure threshold.

Pregnancy and Breast-Feeding

This herb is safe for pregnant and breast-feeding women when consumed appropriately (McGuffin et al., 1997).

SUMMARY OF STUDIES

Keen, H, et al. (1993). This randomized, double-blind, placebo-controlled study included 84 patients with diabetes and neuropathy who took 12 capsules (480 mg of total GLA) over 1 year. Results: Neurological improvements were statistically significant.

Ford et al. (*2001*). A 2-week treatment with evening primrose oil showed improvement in blood flow and nerve function in diabetic rats.

Fukushima et al. (*2001*). Omega-6 and -3 fatty acids, including evening primrose oil, inhibited the increase of serum cholesterol in rats fed a diet with increased cholesterol.

REFERENCES

Belch, J. J., & Hill, A. (2000). Evening primrose oil and borage oil in rheumatologic conditions. *American Journal of Clinical Nutrition, 71*(1 Suppl), 352S–356S.

Blumenthal, M., Goldberg, A., & Brinckmann, J. (Eds.). (2000). *Herbal medicine expanded Commission E monographs.* Austin, TX: American Botanical Council; Newton, MA: Integrative Medicine Communications.

Darlington, L. G., & Stone, T. W. (2001). Antioxidants and fatty acids in the amelioration of rheumatoid arthritis and related disorders. *The British Journal of Nutrition, 85*(3), 251–269.

Ford, I., Cotter, M. A., Cameron, N. E., and Greaves, M. (2001). The effects of treatment with alpha-lipoic acid or evening primrose oil on vascular hemostatic and lipid risk factors, streptozotocin-diabetic rat. *Metabolism, 50*(8), 868–875.

Fukushima, M., Ohhashi, T., Ohno, S., Saitoh, H., Sonoyama, K., Shimada, K., Sekekawa, M., & Nakano, M. (2001).Effects of diets enriched in n-6 or n-3 fatty acids on cholesterol metabolism in older rats chronically fed a cholesterol-enriched diet. *Lipids, 36*(3), 261–266.

Guthrie, D. (August 2000). Herbal approaches to diabetes care. *Advance for Nurse Practitioners,* 56–59.

Hardy, M. L. (2000). Herbs of special interest to women. *Journal of the American Pharmaceutical Association, 40*(2), 234–242.

Horrobin, D. F. (2000). Essential fatty acid metabolism and its modification in atopic eczema. *American Journal of Nutrition, 71*(1 Suppl), 367S–372S.

Keen, H, Payan, J., Allawi, J., Waslker, J., Jamal, G. A., Weir, A. I., Henderson, L. M., Bissessar, E. A., Watkins, P. J., Sampson, M., et al. (1993). Treatment of diabetic neuropathy with gamma-linolenic acid. *Diabetes Care, 16*(1), 8–15.

Kuhn, M. (1999). *Complementary Therapy-Gram* 2(1).

McCaleb, R., Leigh, E., & Morien, K. (2000). *The encyclopedia of popular herbs.* Roseville, CA: Prima Publishing.

McFarlin, B., Gibson, M., O'Rear, J., & Harmon, P. (May–June 1999). A national survey of herbal preparation use by nurse-midwives for labor stimulation: Review of the literature and recommendations for practice. *Journal of Nurse Midwifery, 44*(3), 183–188, 205–216.

McGuffin, M., Hobbs, C., Upton, R., & Goldberg, A. (1997). *Botanical safety handbook.* Boca Raton, FL: CRC Press.

PDR for herbal medicines (1998). Montvale, NJ: Medical Economics Company.

NOTES

NOTES

EVENING PRIMROSE
(Oenothera biennis)

Historical Uses

Evening primrose has been used to treat female complaints, skin problems, and respiratory difficulties.

Growth

Evening primrose is a biennial North American plant with a beautiful, fragrant yellow flower that opens in the evening. It prefers sun and dry soil. The seeds are pressed into oil.

Part Used

• Seed, pressed into oil

Medical Uses

Evening primrose is used for circulation problems caused by diabetes, for symptoms of premenstrual syndrome, and for benign breast pain. It may be beneficial in rheumatic conditions and atopic eczema.

Dosage

Evening primrose oil is standardized to contain 7 to 10 percent gamma-linolenic acid (GLA).

Capsules: 1 to 2 capsules three times daily for premenstrual syndrome, 8 to 12 capsules daily (containing 320–480 mg of total GLA) for diabetic neuropathy, and 6 capsules daily for eczema. Take with meals. It may be several months before an effect is evident.

Warnings

• Evening primrose may cause minor stomach upset, nausea, and headache in large dosages.
• Report side effects to your health-care practitioner.
• Don't take evening primrose with any anti-nausea medications.
• Evening primrose is safe for pregnant and breast-feeding women when consumed appropriately.

FENNEL
(Foeniculum vulgaris)

Historical Uses

Fennel was a sacred herb in medieval times, and bunches of fennel were hung on doors to prevent the effects of witchcraft. Ancient Greeks thought that fennel gave them courage. The Greek meaning of fennel is "to grow thin" (Ody, 1993). In folklore, fennel seeds were used to promote milk flow, help calm colicky babies, suppress appetite, and aid digestion. Fennel has been used in India to aid digestion and freshen breath after eating.

Growth

Fennel is easy to grow from seed; it prefers warm soil with plenty of sun.

Part Used

- Seeds

Major Chemical Compounds

- Volatile oil
- Essential fatty acids
- Flavonoids
- Beta carotene
- Vitamin C
- Calcium
- Iron

Clinical Uses

Traditionally, fennel has been used mainly to aid digestion, relieve stomach spasms, loosen coughs, freshen breath (Tyler, 1993), and promote the flow of breast milk in nursing mothers (Ody, 1993). Fennel water has been given to infants to relieve colic (Tyler, 1993). The German Commission E approved fennel seeds for "dyspepsias, flatulence, catarrh of the upper respiratory tract" (Blumenthal et al., 2000).

Mechanism of Action

Fennel is thought to aid digestion and relieve gas and colic because of the effects of its volatile oils.

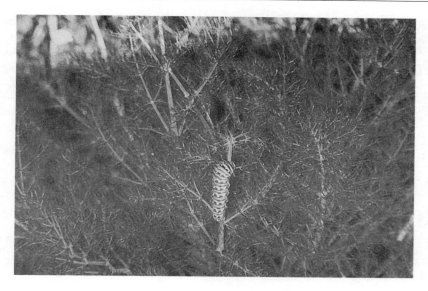

Dosage

Tea by infusion: Place 1 level teaspoon of seeds to 150 mL of boiling water, steep for 5 minutes, strain, and drink 2 to 3 times daily.

Seeds: Up to 1/2 teaspoon of fennel seeds may be chewed after meals. They taste like licorice. The German Commission E limits the use of fennel seeds to 2 weeks (Blumenthal et al., 2000).

Side Effects

Fennel seeds may cause skin irritation and may have a laxative effect.

Contraindications

- High doses of fennel are contraindicated during pregnancy.
- Diabetics who use fennel syrup with honey must consider the sugar content (Blumenthal et al., 2000).

Herb-Drug Interactions

In an animal study, there was a significant interaction between ciprofloxacin and fennel; absorption, distribution, and elimination of ciprofloxacin were all affected. The authors of this study recommended an adequate dosing interval (Zhu et al., 1999).

Pregnancy and Breast-Feeding

Fennel is a uterine stimulant, so high doses should be avoided during pregnancy. Pregnant women may use small amounts in cooking (Ody, 1993). The herb is safe if used in infusions and preparations containing 4 percent essential oil of seeds. It is also safe for use while breast-feeding (Blumenthal et al., 2000; McGuffin et al., 1997).

Pediatric Patients

Fennel syrup and fennel honey may be given to children with upper respiratory infections (Blumenthal et al., 2000).

SUMMARY OF STUDIES

No recent clinical studies in humans are available.

REFERENCES

Blumenthal, M., Goldberg, A., & Brinckmann, J. (Eds.). (2000). *Herbal medicine expanded Commission E monographs* (pp. 126–129). Austin, TX: American Botanical Council; Newton, MA: Integrative Medicine Communications.

McGuffin, M., Hobbs, C., Upton, R., & Goldberg, A. (1997). *Botanical safety handbook* (p. 79). Boca Raton, FL: CRC Press.

Ody, P. (1993). *The complete medicinal herbal.* New York: Dorling Kindersley Publishing.

Tyler, V. (1993). *The honest herbal* (pp. 129–130). Binghamton, NY: Pharmaceutical Products Press.

Zhu, M., Wong, P. Y., & Li, R. C. (1999). Effect of oral administration of fennel (Foeniculum vulgare) on ciprofloxacin absorption and disposition in the rat. *Journal of Pharmacy and Pharmacology, 51*(12), 1391–1396.

NOTES

FENNEL
(Foeniculum vulgaris)

Historical Uses

Fennel was a sacred herb in medieval times, and bunches of fennel were hung on doors to prevent the effects of witchcraft. Ancient Greeks thought that fennel gave them courage. The Greek meaning of fennel is "to grow thin." In folklore, fennel seeds were used to promote milk flow, help calm colicky babies, suppress appetite, and aid digestion. Fennel has been used in India to aid digestion and freshen breath after eating.

Growth

Fennel is easy to grow from seed; it prefers warm soil with plenty of sun.

Part Used

- Seeds

Medical Uses

Traditionally, fennel has been used mainly to aid digestion, relieve stomach spasms, loosen coughs, freshen breath, and promote the flow of breast milk in nursing mothers. Fennel water has been given to infants to relieve colic. Fennel syrup and fennel honey have been used for upper respiratory infections in children.

Dosage

Tea by infusion: Place 1 level teaspoon of seeds to 150 mL of boiling water, steep for 5 minutes, strain, and drink 2 to 3 times daily.

Seeds: Up to 1/2 teaspoon of fennel seeds may be chewed after meals. They taste like licorice. It is recommended that you limit the use of fennel seeds to 2 weeks.

Warnings

- Fennel may cause skin irritation.
- Fennel may have a laxative effect.
- Don't take fennel if you take ciprofloxacin.
- Don't take high doses of fennel during pregnancy because it stimulates the uterus. You may use small amounts in cooking. You may also use infusions and preparations that contain 4 percent essential oil of seeds.
- If you have diabetes and you use fennel syrup or honey, make sure you consider the sugar content.
- Fennel is safe for use while breast-feeding.

RECIPES

Try using dried fennel on grilled fish and in soups, sauces, and stews.

FENUGREEK
(Trigonella foenum-graecum)

Historical Uses

In folklore, fenugreek was said to stimulate milk production and increase appetite. It has been used traditionally to lower blood glucose levels in diabetic patients (Marles & Farnsworth, 1995). In India it has been used as a condiment.

Growth

This annual plant grows in the Mediterranean region.

Part Used

- Seeds

Major chemical compounds

- Steroidal saponins
- Mucilage
- Alkaloid trigonelline
- Flavonoids

Clinical Uses

Fenugreek has been used to lower blood glucose levels in diabetics (Marles & Farnsworth, 1995), to increase fiber in the diet, to reduce inflammation, and to aid digestion. It has also been used for hypercholesterolemia (Sharma et al., 1996; Sowmya & Rajyalakshmi, 1999; Morelli & Zoorob, 2000), hyperlipidemia (Sharma et al., 1996), bronchitis, and loss of appetite. It is approved by the German Commission E for "loss of appetite and external use as a poultice for inflammation" (Blumenthal et al., 2000).

Mechanism of Action

Fenugreek contains soluble fiber that indirectly decreases blood glucose. Its anti-inflammatory and antiviral properties result from fenugreekine (*Natural Medicines*, 2000).

Dosage

Tea: Place 0.5 grams of seeds in 150 mL of cold water, let sit for 3 hours, strain, and drink. Do not exceed 6 grams daily (Blumenthal et al., 2000; *Natural Medicines,* 2000).

Poultice: Prepare a paste of 50 grams of powdered seed in 1 liter of hot water and apply to body part (Blumenthal et al., 2000; *Natural Medicines,* 2000).

Side Effects

External use may cause skin irritation. Two cases of severe allergy to fenugreek have been reported (Patil et al., 1997).

Contraindications

• None are known.

Herb-Drug Interactions

Fenugreek may exaggerate the effects of sulfonylureas or other hypoglycemic agents (*Natural Medicines,* 2000).

Pregnancy and Breast-Feeding

Fenugreek is safe for food use in pregnancy; it should not be used in large amounts because it stimulates the uterus (*Natural Medicines,* 2000). Although it is not recommended during pregnancy, there are no restrictions during breast-feeding (McGuffin et al., 1997).

SUMMARY OF STUDIES

Sowmya & Rajyalakshmi. (*1999*). In this study, 20 adults ages 50 to 65 consumed germinated fenugreek seed powder in doses of 12.5 and 18 grams. Testing of their blood lipid levels after 30 days showed that consumption of 18 grams resulted in a significant reduction in total cholesterol and low-density lipoprotein levels. No significant changes were observed in high-density lipoproteins, very low-density lipoproteins, or triglycerides.

Sharma et al. (*1996*). This 24-week study included 60 patients with type 2 (non–insulin-dependent) diabetes mellitus. Each participant consumed 25 grams of powdered fenugreek seed, divided into two servings and consumed as a soup before lunch and dinner. Results: Serum cholesterol, triglyceride, and low-density lipoprotein levels decreased. High-density lipoprotein levels increased by 10 percent with no adverse effects.

Sharma et al. (*1990*). Use of fenugreek seed powder (50 grams b.i.d.) by insulin-dependent diabetics resulted in reduced fasting blood glucose levels and improved glucose tolerance.

Sur et al. (*2001*). Fenugreek seed extract inhibited tumor cell growth and had a significant anti-inflammatory effect in mice.

Zia et al. (*2001*). Fenugreek showed antiulcer and hypoglycemic actions in mice.

Bordia et al. (*1997*). This was a placebo-controlled study of a combination of fenugreek and ginger in healthy subjects, subjects with coronary artery disease (CAD), and subjects with non–insulin-dependent diabetes mellitus (NIDDM), the last group with or without CAD. The dose was 2.5 grams twice a day for 3 months. In the healthy subjects, there was no effect on blood lipids or blood sugar (fasting and postprandial). In subjects with CAD and NIDDM, fenugreek significantly lowered blood lipids (total cholesterol and triglycerides) without affecting HDL. In subjects with mild NIDDM and no CAD, fasting and postprandial blood sugars decreased significantly. In subjects with severe NIDDM, blood sugar reduction was not significant. Fenugreek did not affect platelet aggregation, fibrinolytic activity, or fibrinogen.

REFERENCES

Blumenthal, M., Goldberg, A., & Brinckmann, J. (Eds.). (2000). *Herbal medicine expanded Commission E monographs.* Austin, TX: American Botanical Council; Newton, MA: Integrative Medicine Communications.

Bordia, A., Verma, S. K., & Srivastava, K. C. (1997). Effect of ginger (*Zingiber officinale Rosc.*) and fenugreek (*Trigonella foenumgraecum L.*) on blood lipids, blood sugar and platelet aggregation in patients with coronary artery disease. *Prostaglandins, Leukotrienes and Essential Fatty Acids, 56*(5), 379–384.

Hoffman, D. (1992). *The new holistic herbal* (p. 200). Boston: Element Books Limited.

Marles, R., & Farnsworth, N. (1995). Antidiabetic plants and their active constituents. *Phytomedicine, 2*(2), 137–189.

McGuffin, M., Hobbs, C., Upton, R., & Goldberg, A. (1997). *Botanical safety handbook.* Boca Raton, FL: CRC Press.

Morelli, V., & Zoorob, R. J. (2000). Alternative therapies: Part II. Congestive heart failure and hypercholesterolemia. *American Family Physician, 62*(6), 1325–1330.

Natural Medicines Comprehensive Database. (2000). *Pharmacist's Letter and Prescriber's Letter* (p. 427). Therapeutic Research Faculty.

Patil, S. P., Niphadkar, P. V., & Bapat, M. M. (1997). Allergy to fenugreek (*Trigonella foenum graecom*). *Annals of Allergy, Asthma and Immunology, 78*(3), 297–300.

Sharma, R., Raghuram, T., & Rao, N. (1990). Effect of fenugreek seeds on blood glucose and serum lipids in type I diabetes. *European Journal of Clinical Nutrition, 44*, 301–306.

Sharma, R., Sarkar, A., Hazra, D., Misra, J., Singh, J., Maheshwari, B., & Sharma, S. (1996).Hypolipidaemic effect of fenugreek seeds: A chronic study in non-insulin dependent diabetic patients. *Phytotherapy Research, 10*, 332–334.

Sowmya, P., & Rajyalakshmi, P. (1999). Hypocholesterolemic effect of germinated fenugreek seeds in human subjects. *Plant Foods Hum Nutr, 53*(4), 359–365.

Sur, P., Das, M., Gomes, A., Vedasiromoni, J. R., Sahu, N. P., Banerjee, S., Sharma, R. M., & Ganguly, D. K. (2001). *Trigonella foenum graecum* (fenugreek) seed extract as an antineoplastic agent. *Phytotherapy Research, 15*(3), 257–259.

Zia, T., Hasnain, S. N., & Hasan, S. K. (2001). Evaluation of the oral hypoglycaemic effect of *Trigonella foenum-graecum L.* (methi) in normal mice. *Journal of Ethnopharmacology, 75*, 191195.

NOTES

FENUGREEK
(Trigonella foenum-graecum)

Historical Uses

In folklore, fenugreek was said to stimulate milk production and increase appetite. It has been used traditionally to lower blood glucose levels in diabetic patients. In India it has been used as a condiment.

Growth

This annual plant grows in the Mediterranean region.

Part Used

• Seeds

Medical Uses

Fenugreek has been used to lower blood glucose levels in diabetics and to lower high cholesterol and blood lipid levels. It has also been used to increase fiber in the diet, to reduce inflammation, and to aid digestion. And it has been used for bronchitis and loss of appetite.

Dosage

Tea: Place 0.5 grams of seeds in 150 mL of cold water, let sit for 3 hours, strain, and drink. Do not exceed 6 grams daily.

Poultice: Prepare a paste of 50 grams of powdered seed in 1 liter of hot water and apply to body part.

Warnings

• External use of fenugreek may cause skin irritation.
• Don't take fenugreek if you take a medication for diabetes.
• If you're pregnant, don't use fenugreek in large amounts because it may stimulate the uterus. Use it only in small amounts in food.
• There are no restrictions during breast-feeding.

FEVERFEW
(Tanacetum parthenium)

Historical Uses

Traditionally, feverfew was used to manage labor pains, to reduce fevers, and to repel insects.

Growth

Feverfew is a member of the daisy family and may be grown in herb gardens in the spring. The plant prefers dry soil and sun.

Part Used

- Leaves

Major Chemical Compounds

- Sesquiterpene lactones, primarily parthenolide

Clinical Uses

Feverfew is used to prevent migraine headaches (Ernst & Pittler, 2000; Palevitch et al., 1997; Murphy et al., 1988; Johnson et al., 1985) and also to treat migraine headaches.

Mechanism of Action

The mechanism by which feverfew works is not fully understood. It may act like non-steroidal anti-inflammatory drugs (NSAIDs) by interfering with the first step of thromboxane synthesis (inhibiting prostaglandin biosynthesis), but it differs from sal-icylates in that it does not inhibit cyclo-oxygenation by prostaglandin synthase (Collier et al., 1980). Feverfew inhibits serotonin release from platelets and polymor-phonuclear leukocyte granules, which benefits patients with migraines or arthritis (*The Lawrence Review of Natural Products,* 1994; Heptinstall et al., 1985). It has shown antinociceptive and anti-inflammatory effects in animals (Jain & Kulkarni, 1999).

Dosage

To be effective at preventing migraines, the parthenolide content of feverfew must be between 0.25 and 0.5 mg. Standardized extract gives 275 mg a day (McCaleb et al., 2000). One study used 100 mg of feverfew leaf (two 50-mg capsules daily). During an acute attack, 1 to 2 grams may be needed. Or two to three leaves may be taken daily with food or juice for migraine or arthritis. It may be 1 to 2 months before an improvement occurs (Ottariano, 1999).

Side Effects

Aphthous ulcerations (mouth sores) have been reported in 12 percent of respondents in a study; these ulcerations are more likely with ingestion of fresh leaves. Feverfew may cause GI upset as well (McGuffin et al., 1997), in addition to an elevated international normalized ratio.

Contraindications

• Feverfew is contraindicated during pregnancy and breast-feeding.

Herb-Drug Interactions

Feverfew should not be taken at the same time as NSAIDs because the herbal effect will be inhibited (Miller L, 1998). Feverfew may decrease platelet aggregation and should not be given with aspirin (Herbst, 1999). Feverfew should not be given to patients who are also taking anticoagulant therapy (Ottariano, 1999).

Pregnancy and Breast-Feeding

Do not use this herb during pregnancy because it may stimulate the uterus and induce abortion (McGuffin et al., 1997). It should not be used during breast-feeding (Ottariano, 1999).

Pediatric Patients

There is no substantial information for children under age 2 (*Natural Medicines*, 2000).

 # SUMMARY OF STUDIES

Palevitch et al. (*1997*). This double-blind, placebo-controlled, crossover study included 57 subjects with severe migraines. The patients took 100 mg of feverfew or placebo daily for 2 months. Results: Feverfew reduced the pain of migraines and improved overall symptoms compared to the placebo; patients in the placebo group experienced increased pain.

Heptinstall et al. (*1992*). The study of three physicochemical assays and bioassay showed parthenolide content and bioactivity. Products varied widely in their parthenolide content, and in some products parthenolide was not detected.

Murphy et al. (*1988*). This randomized, double-blind, placebo-controlled crossover study looked at feverfew for migraine prophylaxis. It included 72 volunteers. Results: Feverfew reduced the mean number and severity of attacks in each 2-month period. It also reduced the degree of vomiting. VAS scores improved. There were no serious side effects.

Johnson et al. (*1985*). This double-blind, placebo-controlled study looked at the efficacy of migraine prophylaxis in 72 volunteers. Results: Feverfew prevented migraine attacks.

Heptinstall et al. (*1985*). Results: Inhibition of granule secretion of platelets and polymorphonuclear leucocytes showed that the pattern of effects of feverfew extracts on platelets is different from that of other inhibitors and that the effect on polymorphonuclear leucocytes is more pronounced than that obtained with very high amounts of nonsteroidal anti-inflammatory drugs.

Collier et al. (*1980*). This study looked at inhibition of prostaglandin biosynthesis by feverfew. Results: Feverfew contains a factor that inhibits prostaglandin biosynthesis, but it differs from that of salicylates in that it does not inhibit cyclo-oxygenation by prostaglandin synthase.

REFERENCES

Awang, D. (1989). Herbal medicine feverfew. *CPJ-RPC, 266–270.*

Collier, H., Butt, N., McDonald-Gibson, & Saeed, S. (October 25, 1980). Extract of feverfew inhibits prostaglandin biosynthesis. *The Lancet, 2*(8200), 922–923.

Ernst, E., & Pittler, M. H. (2000). The efficacy and safety of feverfew (*Tanacetum parthenium L.*): An update of a systemic review. *Public Health Nutrition, 3*(4A), 509–514

Heptinstall, S., Awang, D., Dawson, B., Kindack, D., Knight, D.W., & May, J. (1992). Parthenolide content and bioactivity of feverfew. Estimation of commercial and authenticated feverfew products. *Journal of Pharmacy and Pharmacology, 44*(5), 391–395.

Heptinstall, S., Williamson, L., White, A., & Mitchell, J. (May 11, 1985). Extracts of feverfew inhibit granule secretion in blood platelets and polymorphonuclear leucocytes. *Lancet,* 1071–1073.

Herbst, D. (September 1999). Bad mix. *Natural Health,* 100–103, 147.

Johnson, E., Kadam, N., Hylands, D., & Hylands, P. (1985). Efficacy of feverfew as prophylactic treatment of migraine. *British Medical Journal, 291,* 569–573.

Lawrence Review of Natural Products (1994). Feverfew. Facts and Comparisons. St. Louis, MO.

Jain, N. K., & Kulkarni, S. K. (1999). Antinociceptive and anti-inflammatory effects of *Tanacetum parthenium L.* extract in mice and rats. *Journal of Ethnopharmacology, 68*(1–3), 251–259.

Makheja, A., & Bailey, L. (November 7, 1981). The active principle in feverfew. *The Lancet,* 1054.

McCaleb, R., Leigh, E., & Morien, K. (2000). *The encyclopedia of popular herbs* (pp. 157–152). Roseville, CA: Prima Publishing.

McGuffin, M., Hobbs, C., Upton, R., & Goldberg, A. (1997). *Botanical safety handbook.* Boca Raton, FL: CRC Press.

Miller, L. (1998). Herbal medicinals: Selected clinical considerations focusing on known or potential drug-herb interactions. *Archives of Internal Medicine, 158,* 2200–2211. Cited in Vickers & Zollman (1999). Herbal medicine. *British Medical Journal, 319,* 1050–1053.

Murphy, J., Heptinstall, S., & Mitchell, J. (July 23, 1988). Randomized double-blind placebo-controlled trial of feverfew in migraine prevention. *The Lancet,* 189–192.

Natural Medicines Comprehensive Database. (2000). *Pharmacist's Letter and Prescriber's Letter.* Therapeutic Research Faculty.

Ottariano, S. (1999). *Medicinal herbal therapy: A pharmacist's viewpoint* (pp. 108–110). North Hampton, NH: Nicolin Fields Publishing.

Palevitch, D., Earon, G., & Carosso, R. (1997). Feverfew (*Tanacetum parthenium*) as a prophylactic treatment for migraine: A double-blind-placebo-controlled study. *Phytotherapy Research, 2,* 508–511.

NOTES

NOTES

FEVERFEW
(Tanacetum parthenium)

Historical Uses

Traditionally, feverfew was used to manage labor pains, to reduce fevers, and to repel insects.

Growth

Feverfew is a member of the daisy family and may be grown in herb gardens in the spring. The plant prefers dry soil and sun.

Part used

• Leaves

Clinical Uses

Feverfew is used to prevent and treat migraine headaches.

Dosage

To be effective at preventing migraines, the content of parthenolide (a major chemical component) must be between 0.25 and 0.5 mg. Standardized extract provides 275 mg a day. One study used 100 mg of feverfew leaf (two 50-mg capsules daily). During an acute attack, 1 to 2 grams may be needed. Or two to three leaves may be taken daily with food or juice for migraine or arthritis. It may take 1 to 2 months before an improvement occurs.

Warnings

• Mouth sores were reported by 12 percent of the people who took part in one study; the sores were more likely among people who used fresh leaves.
• Don't take feverfew with nonsteroidal anti-inflammatory drugs (such as ibuprofen, acetaminophen, and so forth), aspirin, or blood thinners.
• Don't take feverfew if you are breast-feeding.

• Feverfew may cause gastrointestinal upset.
• Feverfew may increase the risk of bleeding.
• Don't take feverfew if you are pregnant because it may stimulate the uterus and induce abortion.
• Don't give feverfew to children under age 2.

This information is not intended to be a substitute for qualified medical intervention, counseling, or testing. Talk with your health-care practitioner if you are taking or considering taking any herbal medicine, especially if you are already taking prescription medications. If you experience ANY side effects, stop the herb and report the side effects to your health-care practitioner immediately.

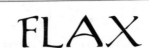

FLAX

⟨Linum usitatissimum⟩

Historical Uses

Flax is one of the earliest foods known to humans. It is also a textile fiber used to make linen. The seed is used in paints (linseed oil). Flax has also been used to make paper (Wood, 1999).

Growth

Flax is cultivated as a crop.

Part Used

- Seeds

Major Chemical Compounds

- Alpha-linolenic acid
- Lignans
- Fiber
- The best source of omega-3 essential fatty acids

Clinical Uses

Flaxseed is used for constipation and for intestinal cleansing in diverticulitis. It is also used for menopausal symptoms and sore throats and for its antioxidant effects. It may help to prevent or decrease the risk of cardiovascular disease (Hasler et al., 2000). Flaxseed is approved by the German Commission E for "chronic constipation, irritable colon, diverticulitis and as mucilage, externally for inflammation" (Blumenthal et al., 2000).

Mechanism of Action

Essential fatty acids reduce the risk of blood clotting and thus decrease the risk of heart disease and stroke. They are building blocks of prostaglandins, which help to reduce pain and inflammation; help promote relaxation in stress; and improve the immune system, skin, and digestive system. Lignans are mildly estrogenic.

Dosage

Flaxseeds: Take 1 tablespoon of flaxseeds (10 g) up to three times a day with a glass of water (at least 150 mL). Flaxseed can be ground, eaten whole, or soaked in water.

Flaxseed oil: Use flaxseed oil to make salad dressings or take 1 to 2 tablespoons a day.

Poultice: Mix flaxseed flour into a paste with warm water and apply poultice to the inflamed area.

To get the best effects from essential fatty acids, it is important to eat a healthy diet that contains vitamins A, B_3, B_6, C, and E; beta carotene; magnesium; selenium; and zinc. Store flaxseed oil in a dark bottle in the refrigerator.

Side effects

None are known.

Contraindications

• Bowel obstruction (McGuffin et al., 1997).

Herb-Drug Interactions

Flaxseed may reduce the absorption of other drugs (Blumenthal et al., 1998; Gruenwald et al., 1998). It should be used cautiously if the patient takes an antidiabetic drug (Blumenthal et al., 1998).

Pregnancy and Breast-Feeding

No restrictions are known (Blumenthal et al., 2000; McGuffin et al., 1997).

 # SUMMARY OF STUDIES

deLorgeril et al. (1994). In the Lyon Diet Heart Study, a 5-year French study, investigators looked at patients who had had a myocardial infarction during the 6 months before the study period. Patients substituted flaxseed spread for butter and also limited their intake of saturated fats. Results: Patients who adopted the study protocol were quite successful in reducing a second myocardial infarction and reducing mortality.

Parbtani & Clark (1996). In this study, patients with systemic lupus erythematosus ate a diet that included 30 grams of flaxseeds a day. Results: Patients had improved kidney function and reduced plasma lipids. (Low-density lipoprotein levels declined by 11 percent.)

Prasad (2001). Secoisolariciresinol diglucoside (SDG), an antioxidant from flaxseed, slowed the development of Type 2 diabetes in rats.

Velasquez & Bhathena (2001). In a review article it was shown that eating flaxseed and soy protein reduced proteinuria and preserved renal function in chronic renal disease in rats. It was unclear which active constituent was responsible.

Kettler (2001). This study showed that use of omega-3 fatty acids, including flaxseeds, may preserve bone density and retard postmenopausal bone loss.

REFERENCES

Blumenthal, M., Busse, W., Goldberg, A., Gruenwald, J., Hall, T., Riggins, C., & Rister, R. (Eds.). (1998). *The complete German Commission E monographs: Therapeutic guide to herbal medicines.* (S. Klein & R. Rister, Trans.). Austin, TX: American Botanical Council; Newton, MA: Integrative Medicine Communications.

Blumenthal, M., Goldberg, A., & Brinckmann, J. (Eds.). (2000). *Herbal medicine expanded Commission E monographs.* Austin, TX: American Botanical Council; Newton, MA: Integrative Medicine Communications.

de Lorgeril, M., Renaud, S., Mamelle, N., et al. (1994). Mediterranean alpha-linolenic acid-rich diet in secondary prevention of coronary heart disease. *The Lancet, 343,* 1454–1459.

Haggerty, W. Flax: Ancient herb and modern medicine. *HerbalGram, 45,* 51–57.

Hasler, C. M., Kundtat, S., & Wool, D. (2000). Functional foods and cardiovascular disease. *Current Atherosclerosis Reports, 2*(6), 467–475.

Kettler, D. B. (2001). Can manipulation of the ratios of essential fatty acids slow the rapid rate of postmenopausal bone loss? *Alternative Medicine Review, 6*(1), 61–77.

McGuffin, M., Hobbs, C., Upton, R., & Goldberg, A. (1997). *Botanical Safety Handbook.* Boca Raton, FL: CRC Press.

Parbtani, A., & Clark (1996). Chapter 17: Flaxseed and its components in renal disease. In *Flaxseed in Human Nutrition* (p. 244). IL:AOCS Press. Cited in W. Haggerty. Flax, ancient herb and modern medicine. *HerbalGram, 45,* 54–55.

PDR for herbal medicines. (1998). Montvale, NJ: Medical Economics Company.

Prasad, K. (2001). Secoisolariciresinol diglucoside (SDG) from flaxseed delays the development of type 2 diabetes in Zucker rat. *Journal of Laboratory and Clinical Medicine, 138*(1), 32–39.

Velasquez, M. T., & Bhathena, S. J. (2001). Dietary phytoestrogens: A possible role in renal disease protection. *American Journal of Kidney Diseases, 37*(5), 1056–1068.

NOTES

FLAX
(Linum usitatissimum)

Historical Uses

Flax is one of the earliest foods known to humans. It is also a textile fiber used to make linen. The seed is used in paints (linseed oil). Flax has also been used to make paper.

Growth

Flax is cultivated as a crop.

Part Used

• Seed

Medical Uses

Flaxseed is used for constipation and for intestinal cleansing in diverticulitis. It is also used for menopausal symptoms and sore throats and for its antioxidant effects.

Dosage

Flaxseeds: Take 1 tablespoon of flaxseeds (10 g) up to three times a day with a glass of water (at least 150 mL). Flaxseed can be ground, eaten whole, or soaked in water.

Flaxseed oil: Use flaxseed oil to make salad dressings or take 1 to 2 tablespoons a day.

Poultice: Mix flaxseed flour into a paste with warm water and apply poultice to the inflamed area.

To get the best effects from essential fatty acids, it is important to eat a healthy diet that contains vitamins A, B_3, B_6, C, and E; beta carotene; magnesium; selenium; and zinc. Store flaxseed oil in a dark bottle in the refrigerator.

Warnings

• Don't take flaxseeds if you have a bowel obstruction.
• If you take any prescription medications, talk with your health-care practitioner before you take flaxseed.
• Don't use flaxseed if you take a medication for diabetes.

RECIPES

Try adding flaxseed, almonds, and raisins to yogurt, or grind some flaxseed and add it to breads or muffins.

FLAXSEED BANANA BREAD

½ cup light brown sugar
1 egg
3 tablespoons oil
1¼ cup unbleached flour
1 teaspoon baking soda
1 cup mashed bananas

½ cup buttermilk (If you don't have buttermilk, place 1 tablespoon of vinegar in low-fat milk)
¾ cup ground flaxseed
1 teaspoon baking powder

Preheat oven to 350°F. In a large bowl, combine sugar, buttermilk, egg, and oil, and beat this mixture together. In a separate bowl, combine flour, flaxseed, baking powder, and soda. Mix these ingredients and add to the other ingredients. Stir, but do not over-mix. Pour into greased loaf pan and bake for about 40 minutes. Cool 5 minutes and, while warm, turn the loaf out onto a rack.

GARLIC

(Allium sativum)

Historical Uses

Called the "stinking rose," garlic has been used by the Egyptians, Chinese, Greeks, Romans, and native North Americans to heal many ailments (Weiss, 1985). In the early 1900s, Dr. W. Minuchin, a physician who was interested in the effects of garlic, performed clinical trials that showed its usefulness in treating tuberculosis, lupus, diphtheria, and infections (Griggs, 1981).

Growth

Plant garlic cloves in the spring, about 2 inches deep and 6 inches apart, in well-drained soil. Planting garlic around vegetable plants helps to repel insects; planting it around fruit and nut trees helps to repel moles (Weiss, 1985). Harvest the garlic when the top of the plant dies.

Part used

• Bulb

Major Chemical Compounds

• Allicin
• Ajoene
• Selenium
• Saponins
• Fructans
• Potassium
• Thiamine
• Calcium
• Magnesium
• Iron
• Phosphorus
• Zinc

Clinical Uses

Garlic is used for hypertension, hypercholesterolemia, infection, and cancer prevention. It is approved by the German Commission E and the World Health Organization for hyperlipidemia and atherosclerotic vascular changes (Blumenthal et al., 2000). It may be useful in mild hypertension (WHO, 1999).

Mechanism of Action

Allicin is a natural antibiotic and antiviral. Ajoene is a platelet aggregation inhibitor. Selenium is a cancer-fighting compound. Saponins lower blood pressure. Fructans stimulate the immune system.

The antibacterial effects of allicin may result from its reducing bacterial conversion of nitrate to nitrite in the stomach, which in turn decreases the formation of carcinogenic nitrosamines (Ernst, 1997). The antibacterial activity and nitrate-scavenging effects of compounds in garlic have been documented in at least 20 studies worldwide, which lends support to the idea of using garlic for infection and cancer prevention (Silagy & Neil, 1994; Amer et al., 1979; Ernst, 1997; Steinmetz et al., 1994; Craig, 1997). Other studies cite the effectiveness of garlic in hypertension and hypercholesterolemia (Koscielny et al., 1999; Silagy & Neil, 1994; Orekov et al., 1994; Warshafsky, 1993; Bordia,1981).

Dosage

Capsules: 600 to 900 mg daily (using a commercial product called Kwai, as was used in the study by Koscielny et al. described under Summary of Studies.).

Fresh garlic: About 4 grams a day.

Allicin is released when garlic is chewed. Its effects are most pronounced when garlic is consumed raw, although it tends to cause halitosis. Also, heat and stomach acid destroy its activity. Enteric-coated tablets are available that release allicin in the small intestine, where it combines with cysteine and is absorbed without causing breath odor (Tyler, 1996).

Side Effects

Side effects are rare at the recommended dosage. Some gastrointestinal upset has been reported. Essential oil of garlic and garlic applied directly to the skin can be irritating. Garlic may increase blood clotting time and elevate international normalized ratios.

Contraindications

- Garlic is contraindicated in patients who are allergic to it.
- Breast-feeding patients should not use garlic.
- Patients should not take large amounts of garlic before undergoing surgery (WHO, 1999).

Herb-Drug Interactions

Garlic should be used cautiously if the patient takes an anticoagulant.

Pregnancy and Breast-Feeding

Garlic is not recommended for pregnant women, breast-feeding mothers, infants of breast-feeding mothers, or small children (McGuffin et al., 1997). Other sources suggest and traditional use states that garlic is safe when consumed in small amounts during pregnancy.

SUMMARY OF STUDIES

Koscielny et al. (1999). This randomized, double-blind, placebo-controlled study included 152 subjects and lasted more than 4 years. The subjects had arterial plaque and a risk factor for heart disease; they consumed either a placebo or Kwai 900 mg. Results: Those who took Kwai had a 2.6 percent reduction in plaque, whereas the placebo group had a 15.6 percent increase in plaque. More benefit was noted in women.

Ernst (1997). This article reviewed 20 epidemiological studies worldwide from 1966 to 1996, 8 studies on garlic, and other studies on onion. Results: A strong association was noted between the consumption of vegetables containing allium and protection against cancer, especially of the gastrointestinal tract.

Silagy & Neil (1994). This meta-analysis included 415 subjects in eight randomized, controlled trials over 4 weeks. Results: Garlic powder preparation of Kwai 600 mg to 900 mg/day may be of some clinical use in patients with mild hypertension. Of seven trials that compared garlic to placebo, three showed a significant reduction in systolic blood pressure and four showed a significant reduction in diastolic blood pressure. The authors felt that more studies were needed.

Steinmetz et al. (1994). This prospective cohort study used the Iowa Women's Health Study of 41,387 women ages 55 to 69. Over the 5-year period in which subjects recorded dietary habits, 212 developed colon cancer. Results: Garlic was the strongest inverse association with risk for colon cancer. No other vegetables containing allium were included in the study.

Orekov et al. (1994). In this in vivo study, blood serum was taken 2 hours after oral administration of a 300-mg garlic powder tablet. Results: Substantially less cholesterol in vivo.

Warshafsky (1993). This meta-analysis of five clinical trials with 365 subjects included four double-blind and all placebo-controlled studies of 8 to 24 weeks. Results: Garlic supplementation of an amount equivalent to one clove a day led to a 9 percent decrease in total serum cholesterol level.

Bordia (1981). This study used two groups with hyperlipidema. Group A had 20 healthy subjects; they were fed 25 mg/kg/day of garlic oil over a 6-month period, followed by 2 months without garlic. Group B had 62 subjects with coronary heart disease and elevated serum cholesterol. Subjects in subgroup B1 received garlic for 10 months. Subjects in subgroup B2 made up the control group. Results: In Group A, garlic significantly lowered serum cholesterol and triglyceride levels (17 and 20 percent) and raised high-density lipoprotein levels (by 29.3 to 41.2 mg/dL). In Group B, garlic decreased serum cholesterol (18 percent), triglyceride, and low-density lipoprotein levels while increasing high-density lipoprotein levels. Conclusion: Essential oil of garlic showed hypolipidemic action in both healthy people and those with coronary artery disease. These changes were not maintained after 2 months without garlic oil.

Amer et al. (1979). In vitro and in vivo animal studies showed topical treatment of fungal infections with garlic produced complete healing in 14 to 17 days following twice-daily application of the extract for 1 week.

Sarrell et al. (2001). In a randomized controlled trial of 103 children aged 6 to 18 years with the diagnosis of otalgia, Otikon, an ear drop containing *Allium sativum* and other herbs, was as effective as anesthetic ear drops.

Kannar et al. (2001). In a double-blind randomized, placebo-controlled study of 46 subjects with hypercholesterolemia, 9.6 mg of an allicin-releasing, enteric-coated garlic supplement over a 12-week period showed a cholesterol-lowering effect.

Lawson et al. (*2001*). From 1989 to 1997 there were many positive studies of the use of garlic to reduce serum cholesterol, but lately these studies have been negated. Lawson et al. reiterate the importance of using a high-quality allicin-releasing garlic supplement as determined under the standardized drug release conditions of U. S. Pharmacopeia Method 724A.

REFERENCES

Amer, M., Taha, M., & Tosson, Z. (1980). The effect of aqueous garlic extract on the growth of dermatophytes. *International Journal of Dermatology, 19*(5), 285–287.

Blumenthal, M., Goldberg, A., & Brinckmann, J. (Eds.). (2000). *Herbal medicine expanded Commission E monographs.* Austin, TX: American Botanical Council; Newton, MA: Integrative Medicine Communications.

Bordia, A. (1981). Effect of garlic on blood lipids in patients with coronary heart disease. *American Journal of Clinical Nutrition, 34,* 100–2103.

Chadha, Y, et al. (Eds.) (1952–1988). *The wealth of India,* 11 volumes. New Delhi: Publications and Information Directorate, CSIR. Cited in M. McGuffin, C. Hobbs, R. Upton, & A. Goldberg.(1997). *Botanical safety handbook* (p. 6). Boca Raton, FL: CRC.

Craig, W. (1997). Phytochemicals: Guardians of our health. *Journal of the American Diet Association, 10* (Suppl 2), S199–204.

Eftekhar, J. (1996). *Garlic: The miracle herb.* FL: Globe.

Ernst, E. (1997). Can allium vegetables prevent cancer? *Phytomedicine, 4*(1), 79–83.

Griggs B. (1981). *Green Pharmacy: The History and Evolution of Western Herbal Medicine.* VT: Healing Arts Press.

Kannar, D., Wattanapenpaiboon, D., Savige, G. S., & Walhquist, M. L. (2001). Hypocholesteremic effect of an enteric-coated garlic supplement. *Journal of American College of Nutrition, 20*(3), 225–231.

Koscielny, J., et al. (1999). The antiatherosclerotic effect of *Allium sativum. Artherosclerosis, 144,* 237–249.

Lawson, L. D., Wang, Z. J., & Papadimitriou, D. (2001). Allicin release under simulated gastrointestinal conditions from garlic powder tablets employed in clinical trials on serum cholesterol. *Planta Medica, 67*(1), 13–18.

Orekhov, A., Tertov, V., Sobenin, I., & Pivovarova, E. (1994). Direct anti-atherosclerosis related effects of garlic. *Annals of Medicine, 27,* 63–65.

Sarrell, E. M., Mandelberg, A., & Cohen, H. A. (2001). Efficacy of naturopathic extracts in the management of ear pain associated with acute otitis media. *Archives of Pediatric and Adolescent Medicine, 155*(7), 796–799.

Silagy, C., & Neil, A. (1994). Garlic as a lipid lowering agent—A meta-analysis. *Journal of Royal College of Physicians London, 28,* 2–8.

Silagy, C., & Neil, A. (1993) A meta-analysis of the effect of garlic on blood pressure. *Journal of Hypertension, 12,* 463–468.

Steinmetz, K., Kushi, L., Bostick, R., Folsum, A., & Potter, J. (1994). Vegetables, fruits, and colon cancer in the Iowa Women's Health Study. *American Journal of Epidemiology, 139,* 1–15.

Tyler, V. (1996). What pharmacists should know about herbal remedies. *Journal of the American Pharmaceutical Association, NS36*(1), 29–37.

Warshafsky, S., Kamer, R., & Sivak, S. (1993). Effect of garlic on total serum cholesterol. *Annals of Internal Medicine, 119*:599–605.

Weiss, G., & Weiss, S. (1985). *Growing and using the healing herbs.* Emmaus, PA: Rodale Press.

World Health Organization. (1999). *WHO monographs on selected medicinal plants.* Vol. 1. Geneva: The Organization.

NOTES

NOTES

GARLIC
(Allium sativum)

Historical Uses

Called the "stinking rose," garlic has been used by the Egyptians, Chinese, Greeks, Romans, and native North Americans to heal many ailments. In the early 1900s, Dr. W. Minuchin, a physician who was interested in the effects of garlic, performed clinical trials that showed the usefulness of garlic in treating tuberculosis, lupus, diphtheria, and infections.

Growth

Plant garlic cloves in the spring, about 2 inches deep and 6 inches apart, in well-drained soil. Planting garlic around vegetable plants helps to repel insects; planting it around fruit and nut trees helps to repel moles. Harvest the garlic when the top of the plant dies.

Part Used

• Bulb

Medical Uses

Garlic is used for high blood pressure, high cholesterol, infections, and cancer prevention.

Dosage

Fresh garlic: About 4 grams a day (preferred over capsules).

Capsules: 600 to 900 mg daily (using a commercial product called Kwai).

Warnings

• Side effects are rare at the recommended dosage. Some gastro-intestinal upset has been reported.
• Garlic may increase the risk of bleeding. Don't take large amounts of before surgery.
• Use garlic cautiously if you take a blood-thinning medication.
• Avoid garlic use in pregnancy. (Some sources and traditional use state that garlic is safe during pregnancy when consumed in small amounts in food.)

• Essential oil of garlic and garlic applied directly to the skin can be irritating.
• Don't take garlic if you are allergic to it.
• Don't use garlic while breast-feeding.
• Garlic is not recommended for breast-feeding infants and small children.

RECIPES

HERB AND GARLIC LINGUINE

1 box light cream cheese
3 tablespoons extra virgin olive oil
1 tablespoon fresh parsley
1 box linguine

¼ cup hot water
1 tablespoon fresh basil
½ tablespoon oregano
4 cloves garlic

Chop garlic cloves into large pieces and simmer in olive oil until warm. At the same time, heat the cream cheese and, when softened, add hot water and whisk. Add the herbs to the cream cheese mixture. Cook the linguine. Strain the garlic out of the oil and add the oil to the linguine. Next, add the cream cheese mixture in the desired amount on top of each plate of linguine. Makes 4 servings.

HEART-HEALTHY GARLIC SPAGHETTI

Using this recipe, I can quickly prepare a healthy meal for my husband and teenage boys even after a long day.

1 box angel hair spaghetti
1 cup olive oil

4–6 cloves garlic
Parmesan cheese

Start boiling the water for the angel hair spaghetti. As it heats, peel and chop the garlic into big chunks. Warm the olive oil and add the garlic. Cook the angel hair, drain, and mix with the garlic oil. Sprinkle with grated parmesan cheese. Enjoy!

GINGER
(Zingiber officinale)

Historical Uses

Greek bakers imported ginger from the Orient to make gingerbread. Spanish mariners brought ginger to the New World.

Growth

Ginger is cultivated in tropical climates.

Part Used

• The knotted and branched rhizome (an underground stem) called the root.

Major Chemical Compounds

• Volatile oils, particularly zingiberene, bisabolene, gingerols, and shogaols
• Niacin
• Vitamin A

Clinical Uses

Ginger is used for nausea and vomiting, motion sickness, and inflammation. It also has anticancer effects (Craig, 1997). Ginger has been shown to relieve nausea and vomiting during pregnancy without adverse effects (Vutyavanich et al., 2001). It is approved by the German Commission E and the World Health Organization (WHO) for "prevention of motion sickness." WHO also has approved ginger for postoperative nausea, pernicious vomiting in pregnancy, and seasickness, whereas the German Commission E approved ginger only for dyspepsia and does not recommend its use during pregnancy (Blumenthal et al., 2000).

Mechanism of Action

Ginger does not influence the inner ear or the oculomotor system; apparently it exerts its antiemetic effect directly on the gastrointestinal system (Holtmann et al., 1989). Anti-inflammatory effects result from inhibition of certain prostaglandins and leukotrienes that cause pain and inflammation, without inhibition of beneficial prostaglandins (McCaleb et al., 2000).

Dosage

The maximum dose of oral ginger is 4 grams of the root per day (*Natural Medicines*, 2000).

Dry ginger root: Studies use 1 gram of dry powdered ginger root. Fresh or freeze-dried ginger root has a better effect.

Capsules: 1 to 2 grams of dry powdered ginger daily in capsule form is equivalent to about 10 grams or ⅓ ounce of fresh ginger root (about a ¼-inch slice). For motion sickness, take 1 gram 30 minutes before a trip; then take 0.5 to 1 gram every 4 to 6 hours to relieve symptoms. Take 500 mg twice a day for headache and pain relief.

Ginger tea: Peel off the outer covering of the ginger root. Cut a ¼-inch slice of ginger and place it in boiling water; simmer for about 10 minutes, and then remove the ginger (Hoffman, 1990). Add honey to taste and sip as needed for nausea.

Crystallized ginger: Available for children.

External use: Ginger may be applied externally as a compress over the abdomen, or ginger oil many be massaged over a painful area to help reduce symptoms of premenstrual syndrome, menstrual cramps, and arthritis. The compress may be made with ginger tea. Use a cloth to absorb the tea, wring it out, and apply the warm cloth to the painful area.

Side Effects

Ginger capsules tend to irritate the stomach and should be taken with food. Ginger may elevate the international normalized ratio.

Contraindications

• Ginger is contraindicated in patients with gallstones (Blumenthal et al., 2000).

Herb-Drug Interactions

Ginger may enhance the effects of anticoagulants (McCaleb et al., 2000).

Pregnancy and Breast-Feeding

Ginger is not approved for morning sickness during pregnancy (McGuffin et al., 1997; Blumenthal et al., 2000), although traditional evidence and a study on hyperemesis gravidarum (Fisher-Rasmussen et al., 1990) suggest that it is safe at an appropriate dosage.

SUMMARY OF STUDIES

Bone, Wilkinson, Young, & McNeil (1990). This double blind, randomized study looked at the effects of ginger root on postoperative nausea and vomiting in 60 women who had major gynecological surgery. Results: 1 gram of powered ginger root significantly reduced the incidence of postoperative emetic sequelae in comparison to placebo, and had the same effect as metoclopramide.

Fischer-Rasmussen, Kjaer, Dahl, & Asping (1990). This double-blind, randomized, cross-over trial included 30 women with hyperemesis gravidarum. Results: 1 gram of powered ginger root was better than placebo in lessening or eliminating the symptoms of hyperemesis gravidarum.

Holtmann, Clarke, Scherer, & Hohn (1989). This controlled, double-blind study of 38 male and female subjects ages 22 to 34 looked at the anti-motion sickness mechanism of ginger. Results: Any reduction of motion-sickness symptoms results from the effect of ginger root on the gastric system and not from a CNS mechanism.

Aksel, Brask, Kambskand, & Hentzer (1988). This double-blind, randomized, placebo-controlled study of 80 naval cadets used ginger root against seasickness. Results: Powered ginger root reduced the tendency toward vomiting and cold sweating significantly more than placebo.

Mowrey & Clayson (1982). This randomized, placebo-controlled study of motion sickness included 36 male and female undergraduates. Results: Powered ginger root was superior to Dramamine in reducing motion sickness.

Vutyavanich et al. (2001). In a trial of randomized controlled, double-masked design, 70 pregnant women took either oral ginger, 1 gram per day, or placebo for 4 days. Results showed that ginger was effective in relieving nausea and vomiting in pregnancy without adverse effects.

Power et al. (2001). In a survey of 488 obstetricians/gynecologists concerning management of nausea and vomiting in pregnancy, 51.8 percent recommended taking ginger.

REFERENCES

Aksel, G., Brask, T., Kambskard, J., & Hentzer, E. (1988). Ginger root against seasickness. *Acta Otolaryngology, 105,* 45–49.

Backon, J. (1986). Ginger. Inhibition of thromboxane synthetase and stimulation of prostacyclin: Relevance for medicine and psychiatry. *Medical Hypotheses, 20,* 271–278.

Blumenthal, M., Goldberg, A., & Brinckmann, J. (Eds.). (2000). *Herbal medicine expanded Commission E monographs* (pp. 153–159). Austin, TX: American Botanical Council; Newton, MA: Integrative Medicine Communications.

Bone, M., Wilkinson, D., Young, J., & McNeil, J. (1990). Ginger root—A new antiemetic. The effect of ginger root on postoperative nausea and vomiting after major gynaecological surgery. *Anaesthesia, 45,* 669–671.

Craig, W. (1997). Phytochemicals: Guardians of our health. *Journal of the American Diet Association, 10* (Suppl 2), S199–204.

Fisher-Rasmussen, W., Kjaer, S., Dahl, C., & Asping, U. (1990). Ginger treatment of hyperemesis gravidarum. *Euopean Journal of Obstetrics, Gynecology, and Reproductive Biology, 38,* 19–24.

Holtmann, S., Clarke, A., Scherer, H., & Hohn, M. (1989). The anti-motion sickness mechanism of ginger. *Acta Oto-Laryngologica, 108,* 168–174.

McCaleb, R., Leigh, E., & Morien, K. (2000). *The Encyclopedia of Popular Herbs.* Roseville, CA: Prima Publishing.

McGuffin, M., Hobbs, C., Upton, R., & Goldberg, A. (1997). *American Herbal Society's Botanical Safety Handbook* (p. 125). Florida: CRC Press.

Mowrey, D., & Clayson, D. (March 20, 1982). Motion sickness, ginger, and psychophysics. *The Lancet*, 655–657.

Natural Medicines Comprehensive Database. (2000). *Pharmacist's Letter and Prescriber's Letter*. Therapeutic Research Faculty.

Power, M. L., Holzman, G. , & Schulkin, J. (2001). A survey on the management of nausea and vomiting in pregnancy by obstetrician/gynecologists. *Primary Care Update Obstetrics and Gynecology, 8*(2), 69–72.

Vutyavanich, T., Kraisarin, T., & Ruangari, R. (2001). Ginger for nausea and vomiting in pregnancy: Randomized, double-masked, placebo-controlled trial. *Obstetrics and Gynecology, 97*(4), 577–582.

NOTES

GINGER
(Zingiber officinale)

Historical Uses

Greek bakers imported ginger from the Orient to make gingerbread. Spanish mariners brought ginger to the New World.

Growth

Ginger is cultivated in tropical climates.

Part Used

• The knotted and branched rhizome (an underground stem) called the root.

Medical Uses

Ginger is used for nausea and vomiting, motion sickness, and inflammation. It may help to prevent cancer.

Dosage

Maximum dose of oral ginger is 4 grams of the root per day.

Dry ginger root: Studies use 1 gram of dry powdered ginger root. Fresh or freeze-dried root has a better effect.

Capsules: 1 to 2 grams dry powdered ginger daily in capsule form is equivalent to about 10 gram or $1/3$ of an ounce of fresh ginger root (about a $1/4''$ slice). For motion sickness, take 1 gram 30 minutes before a trip; then take 0.5 to 1 gram every 4 to 6 hours to relieve symptoms. Take 500 mg twice a day for headache and pain relief.

Ginger tea: Peel off the outer covering of the ginger root. Cut a $1/4''$ slice of ginger and place it in boiling water; simmer for about 10 minutes and then remove the ginger. Add honey to taste, and sip as needed for nausea, fever, sore throat, congestion, flu, and chemotherapy side effects.

Crystallized ginger: Available for children.

External use: Ginger may be applied externally as a compress over the abdomen, or ginger oil many be massaged over a painful area to help reduce symptoms of premenstrual syndrome, menstrual cramps, and arthritis. The compress may be made with tea. Use a cloth to absorb the tea, wring it out, and apply the warm cloth to the painful area.

Warnings

- Ginger capsules tend to irritate the stomach and should be taken with food.
- Ginger may increase the risk of bleeding. Consult your health-care practitioner if you take a blood-thinning medication.
- Don't take ginger if you have gallstones.
- Ginger is not approved for morning sickness during pregnancy.

GINKGO
(Ginkgo biloba)

Historical Uses

Legend has it that Chinese monks saved the ginkgo tree from extinction by growing it in monastery gardens (McCaleb et al., 2000).

Growth

The ginkgo is the oldest known living tree in the world. It is not difficult to grow, and ginkgo trees can be found in many city areas in the United States, including Central Park in New York City. The trees are able to withstand pollution and disease. Their leaves turn yellow in the fall.

Part Used

• Dried leaves

Major Chemical Compounds

• Diterpenes known as ginkgolides, sesquiterpene bilobalide, quercetin

Clinical Uses

Ginkgo is used for peripheral vascular disease, such as intermittent claudication and cerebral insufficiency. It is approved by the German Commission E and the World Health Organization (Blumenthal et al., 2000). *Ginkgo biloba* is licensed in Germany for treating cerebral dysfunction with difficulties in memory, dizziness, tinnitus, headaches, emotional instability with anxiety, and intermittent claudication (Kleinman & Knipschild, 1992). Its antistress effect makes *ginkgo biloba* useful in the treatment of Alzheimer's disease (DeFeudis & Drieu, 2000). It helps to improve memory (Stough et al., 2001) and may be useful in reducing symptoms of attention deficit hyperactivity disorder (ADHD) (Lyon et al., 2001).

Mechanism of Action

Diterpenes known as ginkgolides combine with a sesquiterpene bilobalide in *Ginkgo biloba* extract to improve the tolerance of brain tissue to hypoxia and to increase cerebral circulation (DeFeudis & Drieu, 2000). Rutin-type flavones reduce capillary fragility, tend to prevent ischemic brain damage, and inhibit lipid peroxidation of cell membranes by inactivating free oxygen radicals. These effects combine to alleviate impaired cerebral circulation, particularly in elderly people, and relieve unpleasant associated symptoms,

131

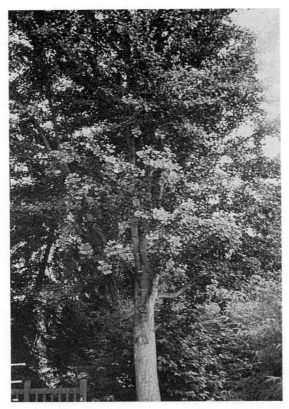

such as dizziness, depression, tinnitus, and short-term memory loss (Tyler, 1996). *Ginkgo biloba* extract (Egb 761) helps in neurodegenerative disorders because of its antioxidant properties and enhances "neuronal plasticity" (DeFeudis & Drieu, 2000).

Dosage

Standardized extract: For people over age 50, studies have used 120 to 240 mg daily in divided doses for 4 weeks to 9 months. It takes 4 to 6 weeks for positive effects to occur. The patient should be reviewed at 3 months. Standardized products used in studies include Schwabe Egb 761 extract, BioGinkgo, and Whole Foods Ginkgo. Extract of *Ginkgo biloba* used in studies and known as Egb is standardized to 24 percent flavone glycosides and 6 percent terpenes. In a review of the literature, Egb showed a higher rate of treatment response at 240 mg per day than at 120 mg per day without increasing side effects (LeBars & Kastelan, 2000).

Side Effects

Ginkgo biloba may elevate the international normalized ratio. It also may cause mild gastrointestinal disturbances, allergic skin reactions, and headache. If headache occurs, the herb should be discontinued.

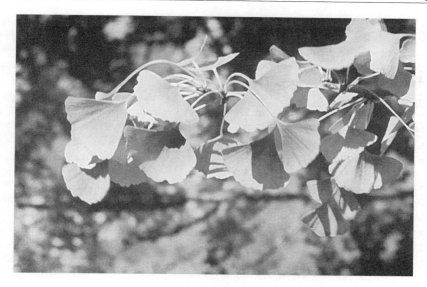

Contraindications

• None are known.

Herb-Drug Interactions

Ginkgo may interact with trazodone (Desyrel), causing CNS depression and coma (Natural Medicines, September 2000). It may increase bleeding times when taken with aspirin (Rosenblatt, 1997) or Coumadin (Herbst, 1999; Miller, 1998). Also, it may potentiate the effects of papaverine in treating male impotence (Sikora et al., 1989).

Pregnancy and Breast-Feeding

No restrictions are known.

SUMMARY OF STUDIES

Oken et al. (1998). This meta-analysis of 4 studies included 212 patients who used standardized extract (50:1), standardized to 6 percent terpene lactones and 24 percent ginkgo flavone glycosides. Products included Tebonin (Egb 761, Schwabe of Germany) and Kaveri (LI 1440, Lichtwer Pharma of Berlin and Pittsburgh). Results: 120 to 240 mg *Ginkgo biloba* leaf extract for 3 to 6 months had a small but significant effect on objective measures of cognitive function in Alzheimer's disease without causing adverse effects.

Roncin et al. (1996). This placebo-controlled clinical trial included 44 mountain climbers, half of whom took 80 mg of standardized ginkgo extract twice daily; the others took a placebo. Results: Ginkgo was dramatically effective in preventing altitude sickness and was more effective than placebo in preventing cold-related circulation problems.

Le Bars et al. (*1997*). This placebo-controlled, double-blind, randomized trial included 202 subjects and lasted 52 weeks. The subjects used an extract of *Ginkgo biloba* (Schwabe's Egb 761), known in the United States as Ginkoba or Ginkgold at a dosage of 40 mg t.i.d. before meals for dementia. Results: A slight improvement in outcomes with mild to moderate gastrointestinal symptoms.

Kanowski et al. (*1996*). This double-blind, placebo-controlled, randomized, 24-week study included 156 men and women with Alzheimer's disease and multi-infarct dementia. They received *Ginkgo biloba* at a dosage of 120 mg b.i.d. Results: Improvement was noted in psychiatric tests and mild depressive symptoms compared to placebo.

Hofferberth (*1994*). This double-blind, placebo-controlled, 12-week study included 40 patients with Alzheimer's disease who took 80 mg of ginkgo (Egb 761) or placebo t.i.d. Results: Memory and attention improved significantly after one month. Psychopathology, psychomotor performance, functional dynamics, and neurophysiology improved as well. No side effects were noted.

Schubert & Halama (*1993*). This double-blind, placebo-controlled, randomized, 8-week study included 40 subjects ages 51 to 78 with resistant depression. These patients showed insufficient response to tricyclic and tetracyclic antidepressants for 3 months. Patients continued on their medications and also received either 80 mg of ginkgo t.i.d. or a placebo. Results: Improvement was noted in depressive symptoms after 4 weeks, with a highly significant improvement after 8 weeks and a significant improvement in cognitive function in the ginkgo group.

Stough et al. (*2001*). In a randomized, double-blind, placebo-controlled clinical trial of 61 subjects using *Ginkgo biloba* extract (Egb) over 30 days, resuslts showed a significant improvement in working memory.

Lyon et al. (*2001*). In an open study of 36 children with ADHD using AD-FX of CV Technologies (a combination herbal product *containing* American ginseng extract [*Panax quinquefolium*] 200 mg and *Ginkgo biloba* extract 50 mg), results showed improvement in symptoms after 2 and 4 weeks of treatment.

Zhang et al. (*2000*). *Ginkgo biloba* extract (Egb 761) was shown to help regulate hypertension and protect cerebral microcirculation in rats.

Wesnes et al. (*2000*). A double-blind, placebo-controlled, 14-week, parallel group multicenter trial of two dosing regimens of capsules containing standardized extracts of *Ginkgo biloba* (GK501) and *Panax ginseng* (G115) 100 mg in 256 healthy subjects showed that the combination extracts improved working and long-term memory in a 12-week period, including a 2-week washout period (2 weeks without taking the herb).

REFERENCES

Blumenthal, M., Goldberg, A., & Brinckmann, J. (Eds.). (2000). *Herbal medicine expanded Commission E monographs* (pp. 160–169, 486). Austin, TX: American Botanical Council; Newton, MA: Integrative Medicine Communications.

DeFeudis, F. V., & Drieu, K. (2000). *Ginkgo biloba* extract (Egb 761) and CNS functions: Basic studies and clinical applications. *Current Drug Targets, 1*(1), 25–28.

Foster, S. (March 1996). Ginkgo biloba. *Herbs for Health*, 30–33.

Herbst, D. (September 1999,). Bad mix. *Natural Health,* 100–103, 147.

Hofferberth, B. (1994). The efficacy of EGb 761 in patients with senile dementia of the Alzheimer type, a double-blind, placebo-controlled study on different levels of investigation. *Human Psychopharmacology, 9,* 215–222.

Kanowski, D., Herrmann, W. M., Stephan, K., Wierich, W., & Horr, R. (1996). Proof of efficacy of the *Ginkgo biloba* special extract Egb 761 in outpatients suffering from mild to moderate primary degenerative dementia of the Alzheimer type or multi-infarct dementia. *Pharmacopsychiatry, 29,* 47–56.

Kleinjen, J., & Knipschild, P. (1992). Ginkgo biloba. *The Lancet, 340,* 1136–1139.

Le Bars, P. L. (1997). A placebo-controlled, double-blind, randomized trial of an extract of Ginkgo biloba for dementia. *Journal of the American Medical Association, 278*(16), 1327–1332.

LeBars, P. L., & Kastelan, J. (2000). Efficacy and safety of a *Ginkgo biloba* extract. *Public Health Nutrition, 3*(4A), 495–499.

Lyon, M. R., Cline, J. C., Totosy de Zepetnek, J., Shan, J. J., Pang, P., & Benishin, C. (2001). Effect of the herbal extract combination *Panax quinquefolium* and *Ginkgo biloba* on attention-deficit hyperactivity disorder: A pilot study. *Journal of Psychiatry and Neuroscience, 26(3), 221–228.*

McCaleb, R., Leigh, E., & Morien, K. (2000). *The Encyclopedia of Popular Herbs.* Roseville, CA: Prima Publishing.

Miller, L. (1998). Herbal medicinals: Selected clinical considerations focusing on known or potential drug-herb interactions. *Archives of Internal Medicine, 158,* 2200–2211. Cited in Vickers & Zollman (1999). Herbal medicine. *British Medical Journal, 319,* 1050–1053.

Mouren, X., Caillard, P., & Schwartz, F. (1994). Study of the anti-ischemic action of Egb761 in the treatment of peripheral arterial occlusive disease by TcPO2 determination. *Angiology, 45,* 413–417.

Oken, B. S., Storzbach, D. M., & Kaye, J. A. (1998). The efficacy of *Ginkgo biloba* on cognitive function in Alzheimer disease. *Archives of Neurology, 55,* 1409–1415.

Prescriber's Letter (September 2000). Neurology/psychiatry (p. 53). Therapeutic Research Faculty.

Roncin, J., Schwartz, F., & D'Arbigny, P. (1996). Egb 761 in control of acute mountain sickness and vascular reactivity to cold exposure. *Aviation Space and Environmental Medicine, 67*(5), 445–452.

Rosenblatt, M., & Mindel, J. (1997). Spontaneous hyphema associated with ingestion of Ginkgo biloba extract [letter]. *New England Journal of Medicine, 336*(15), 1108.

Schubert, H, & Halama, P. (1993). Depressive episode primarily unresponsive to therapy in elderly patients: Efficacy of *Ginkgo biloba* extract (Egb 761) in combination with antidepressants. *Geriatr Forsch, 3,* 45–53.

Sikora, R., Sohn, M., Deutz, F., et al. (1989). *Ginkgo biloba* extract in the therapy of erectile dysfunction [abstract]. *Journal of Urology, 141,* 188A.

Stough, C., Clarke, J., Lloyd, J., & Nathan, P. J. (2001). Neuropsychological changes after 30-day *Ginkgo biloba* administration in healthy participants. *International Journal of Neuropsychopharmacology, 4*(2), 131–134.

Tyler, V. (1996). What pharmacists should know about herbal remedies. *Journal of the American Pharmaceutical Association, NS36*(1), 29–37.

Wesnes, K. A., Ward, T., McGinty, A., & Petrini, O. (2000). The memory enhancing effects of a *Ginkgo biloba/Panax ginseng* combination in healthy middle-aged volunteers. *Psychopharmacology (Berlin), 152*(4), 353–361.

Zhang, J., Fu, S., Liu, S., Mao, T., & Xiu, R. (2000). The therapeutic effect of *Ginkgo biloba* extract in SHR rats and its possible mechanisms based on cerebral microvascular flow and vasomotion. *Clinical Hemorheology and Microcirculation, 23*(2–4), 133–138.

NOTES

GINKGO
(Ginkgo biloba)

Historical Uses

Legend has it that Chinese monks saved the ginkgo tree from extinction by growing it in monastery gardens.

Growth

Ginkgo is the oldest known living tree in the world. It is not difficult to grow, and ginkgo trees can be found in many city areas in the United States, including Central Park in New York City. The trees are able to withstand pollution and disease. Their leaves turn yellow in the fall.

Part Used

• Dried leaves

Medical Uses

Ginkgo is used for circulation problems, Alzheimer's disease, difficulties with memory, ringing in the ears, headaches, and dizziness. *Ginkgo biloba* is licensed in Germany for treating: cerebral dysfunction with difficulties in memory, dizziness, tinnitus (ringing in the ears), headaches, emotional instability with anxiety, and intermittent claudication.

Dosage

Standardized extract: For people over age 50, studies have used 120 to 240 mg daily in divided doses for 4 weeks to 9 months. It takes 4 to 6 weeks for positive effects to occur. Dosage and effects should be reviewed in 3 months. Standardized products used in studies include Schwabe Egb 761 extract, BioGinkgo, and Whole Foods Ginkgo. Extract of *Ginkgo biloba* used in studies and known as Egb is standardized to 24 percent flavone glycosides and 6 percent terpenes.

Warnings

• *Ginkgo biloba* may increase the risk of bleeding.
• It may cause mild stomach disturbances, allergic skin reactions, and headache. If you get a headache, stop taking the herb and consult your health-care practitioner.
• Don't take *Ginkgo biloba* if you take trazodone (Desyrel), aspirin, a blood thinner, or papaverine.

This information is not intended to be a substitute for qualified medical intervention, counseling, or testing. Talk with your health-care practitioner if you are taking or considering taking any herbal medicine, especially if you are already taking prescription medications. If you experience ANY side effects, stop the herb and report the side effects to your health-care practitioner immediately.

GINSENG
(Panax ginseng)

Historical Uses

Ginseng has been used medicinally in Asia for more than 5000 years (McCaleb et al., 2000). It is known as the ruler of tonic herbs. It is also known as "root of man."

Growth

This perennial plant is indigenous to China and is cultivated in many countries.

Part Used

• Root

Major Chemical Compounds

• Triterpenoid saponins, especially ginsenosides (Hou, 1977).

Clinical Uses

Ginseng is approved by the German Commission E and the World Health Organization for use as an adaptogenic (for stress), an anti-fatigue agent, an anti-stress agent, and a tonic (Blumenthal et al., 2000). In Germany, ginseng may be labeled as an aid to convalescence and a tonic to treat fatigue, reduced work capacity, and poor concentration (Foster, 1999).

Mechanism of Action

Triterpenoid saponins are believed to help the body build vitality, resist stress, and overcome disease. Ginseng inhibits platelet aggregation by inhibiting thromboxane A2 production (Park et al., 1995). Ginsenosides may act on the pituitary gland, not the adrenal glands. The pituitary secretes corticosteroids indirectly through the release of adrenocorticotrophic hormone and also stimulates nerve fibers in the cerebral cortex (Foster, 1999). Ginseng may lower blood glucose levels (Marles & Farnsworth, 1995).

Dosage

The dosage depends on the ginsenoside content and should start at the lowest level possible. Use a standardized product. The typical dosage of product containing 5 percent ginsenosides is 200 mg taken one to three times daily. For long-term use, the patient should take ginseng in cycles of 15 to 20 days on and then 2 weeks off.

Side Effects

Studies using standardized extracts report no side effects. One older study reported hypertension, euphoria, nervousness, insomnia, skin eruptions, and morning diarrhea. Women taking ginseng may experience breast tenderness and may need to reduce the dosage. An estrogenizing effect was noted in studies of male animals (Murray, 1995, p. 277; Kanowski et al., 1996). Ginseng may elevate the international normalized ratio.

Contraindications

• Ginseng is contraindicated in patients with hypertension (McGuffin et al., 1997).

Herb-Drug Interactions

Ginseng should not be taken with insulin, sulphonylureas, or biguanides (Miller, 1998). Taking ginseng with phenelzine sulphate or a monoamine oxidase inhibitor may cause headache, tremulousness, or manic episodes (Miller, 1998). Taking it with estrogens or corticosteroids may have additive effects (Miller, 1998). Ginseng may intensify or interfere with digoxin (Miller, 1998). It may alter bleeding time when taken with anticoagulants (Miller, 1998).

Pregnancy and Breast-Feeding

Use of ginseng during pregnancy and breast-feeding is controversial.

 # SUMMARY OF STUDIES

Hallstrom et al. (1982). This double-blind, crossover, placebo-controlled, 2-week study included 12 nurses who were changing shifts from day to night. Results: Taking 1 to 2 grams of Korean ginseng produced higher scores of competence, mood, and physical performance compared with placebo. Ginseng lowered blood glucose levels.

D'Angelo et al. (1986). This double-blind, crossover study of university students showed that ginseng increased psychomotor function and well-being.

Wesnes et al. (2000). A double-blind, placebo-controlled, 14-week, parallel group multicenter trial of two dosing regimens of capsules containing standardized extracts of *Ginkgo biloba* (GK501) and *Panax ginseng* (G115) 100 mg in 256 healthy subjects showed that the combination extracts improved working and long-term memory in a 12-week period, including a 2-week washout period.

REFERENCES

Blumenthal, M., Goldberg, A., & Brinckmann, J. (Eds.). (2000). *Herbal medicine expanded Commission E monographs* (pp. 170–177). Austin, TX: American Botanical Council; Newton, MA: Integrative Medicine Communications.

D'Angelo, L., Grimaldi, R., Caravaggi, M., Marcoli, M., Perucea, E., Lecchini, Frigo, G. M., & Crema, A. A double-blind, placebo controlled clinical study on the effect of a standardized ginseng extract on psychomotor performance in healthy volunteers. *Journal of Ethnopharmacology, 16,* 15–22.

Foster, S. (May/June 1999). Stress less. *Herbs for Health,* 38–42.

Hallstrom, C., Fulder, S., & Carruthers, M. (1982). Effect of ginseng on the performance of nurses on night duty. *Complementary Medicine East and West, 6,* 277–282.

Hou, J. P. (1977). The chemical constituents of ginseng plants. *Complementary Medicine East and West, 5*(2), 123–145.

Kanowski, S., et al. (1996). Proof of efficacy of the *Gingko biloba* special extract Egb 761 in outpatients suffering from mild to moderate primary degenerative dementia of the Alzheimer type or multi-infarct dementia. *Pharmacopsychiatry, 29,* 47–56.

Marles, R., & Farnsworth, N. (1995). Antidiabetic plants and their active constituents. *Phytomedicine, 2*(2), 137–189.

McCaleb, R., Leigh, E., & Morien, K. (2000). *The Encyclopedia of Popular Herbs.* Roseville, CA: Prima Publishing.

McGuffin, M., Hobbs, C., Upton, R., & Goldberg, A. (1997) *Botanical Safety Handbook.* New York: CRC.

Miller, L. (1998). Herbal medicinals: Selected clinical considerations focusing on known or potential drug-herb interactions. *Archives of Internal Medicine, 158,* 2200–2211. Cited in Vickers & Zollman (1999). Herbal medicine. *British Medical Journal, 319,* 1050–1053.

Murray, M. (1995). *The Healing Power of Herbs.* Roseville, CA: Prima Publishing.

Park, H., Rhee, M. H., Park, K. M., Nam, K. Y., & Park, K. H. (1995). Effect of non-saponin fraction from *Panax ginseng* on cGMP and thromboxane A2 in human platelet aggregation. *Journal of Ethnopharmacology, 49,*157–62 [Medline].

Tyler, V. (1993). *The honest herbal.* Binghamton, NY: Pharmaceutical Products Press.

Wesnes, K. A., Ward, T., McGinty, A., & Petrini, O. (2000). The memory enhancing effects of a *Ginkgo biloba/Panax ginseng* combination in healthy middle-aged volunteers. *Psychopharmacology (Berlin), 152*(4), 353–361.

NOTES

GINSENG
(Panax ginseng)

Historical Uses

Ginseng has been used medicinally in Asia for more than 5000 years. It is known as the ruler of tonic herbs. It is also known as "root of man."

Growth

This perennial plant is indigenous to China and is cultivated in many countries.

Part Used

• Root

Medical Uses

Ginseng is used as an adaptogenic (for stress), an anti-fatigue agent, an anti-stress agent, and a tonic.

Dosage

The dosage depends on the ginsenoside content and should start at the lowest level possible. Use a standardized product. The typical dosage of product containing 5 percent ginsenosides is 200 mg taken one to three times daily. During long-term use, take ginseng in cycles of 15 to 20 days on and then 2 weeks off.

Warnings

• Ginseng may cause high blood pressure, nervousness, insomnia, skin eruptions, and morning diarrhea.
• Women taking ginseng may experience breast tenderness. If you develop this side effect, reduce the dosage.
• Ginseng may increase the risk of bleeding.
• Don't take ginseng if you have high blood pressure.
• Don't use ginseng if you take phenelzine sulphate, an MAO inhibitor (a type of anti-depressant), estrogen (as in hormone replacement therapy), a corticosteroid, digoxin, an anticoagulant (blood thinner), insulin, or an oral antidiabetic medication.
• Use of ginseng is controversial during pregnancy or breast-feeding. Talk with your health-care practitioner.

RECIPE

CHICKEN GINSENG SOUP

Try adding 1 ounce of *Panax ginseng* to a pot of chicken soup. It is great during the winter when stress is high.

142

GOLDENSEAL
(Hydrastis canadensis)

Historical Uses

Sometimes called "poor man's ginseng," goldenseal was discovered by Cherokee Indians who used it for eyewashes, acne, and eczema. The Food and Agriculture Organization of the United Nations cites goldenseal as one of the best-selling herbs internationally (Bannerman,1997). It is very bitter.

Growth

Goldenseal is found in wooded areas in eastern North America, but it is endangered because of overharvesting. The plant prefers moist soil and shade.

Part Used

• Root

Major Chemical Compounds

• Alkaloids of berberine and hydrastine

Clinical Uses

Goldenseal is used for infections of the mucous membranes, digestive disorders, gastritis, peptic ulcers, colitis, and traveler's diarrhea. It has been used to treat streptococcus, staphylococcus, and bacterial vaginosis. Werbach and Murray (1994) note that goldenseal's major constituent (berberine) has also been effective in treating candidiasis. Scientists have disproved the rumor that goldenseal masks morphine in urine testing (Foster & Duke, 1990).

Mechanism of Action

Berberine has antibacterial, antifungal, and antiprotozoal properties and is bacteriostatic for streptococci (Werbach & Murray, 1994; *Alternative Medicine Review,* 2000). Berberine is responsible for the yellow color of goldenseal.

Dosage

Use standardized extract of 5 percent to 15 percent berberine.

Capsules: 250 to 500 mg three times a day. Combination products that contain goldenseal should be taken four times a day. Use goldenseal for only 1 week because it disrupts intestinal flora. A dose of *Lactobacillus acidophilus* should be given with goldenseal because it is a helpful bacteria for the intestine (Ottariano, 1999).

Side Effects

Goldenseal may interfere with vitamin B metabolism. The German Commission E has noted significant nausea, vomiting, diarrhea, and respiratory and cardiac depression in dogs and cats given high doses (25 mg/kg) of goldenseal (Chichon, 2000). Goldenseal may lower blood glucose levels.

Contraindications

• Goldenseal is contraindicated during pregnancy.

Herb-Drug Interactions

None are known.

Pregnancy and Breast-Feeding

Goldenseal should not be used by pregnant women because it has uterine stimulant effects (Blumenthal et al., 1998; McGuffin et al., 1997). It also should not be used during breast-feeding.

SUMMARY OF STUDIES

Govindan & Govindan (2000). Ten samples of goldenseal were analyzed by thin-layer chromatography. Only five contained both hydrastine and berberine; four contained berberine; and one did not contain either of the alkaloids.

REFERENCES

Alternative Medicine Review (2000). Berberine. 5(2), 175–177.

Bannermann, J. (1997). Goldenseal in world trade: Pressures and potentials. *HerbalGram, 41,* 51–52.

Blumenthal, M., Busse, W., Goldberg, A., Gruenwald, J., Hall, T., Riggins, C., & Rister, R. (Eds.). (1998). *The complete German Commission E monographs: Therapeutic guide to herbal medicines.* (S. Klein & R. Rister, Trans.). Austin, TX: American Botanical Council; Newton, MA: Integrative Medicine Communications.

Chichon, P. (August 2000). Herbs and the common cold. *Advance for Nurse Practitioners,* 31–32.

Foster, S., & Duke, J. (1990). *Eastern/central medicinal plants.* New York: Houghton Mifflin.

Govindan, M., & Govindan, G. (2000). A convenient method for the determination of the quality of goldenseal. *Fitoterapia,* 71(3), 232–235.

McGuffin, M., Hobbs, C., Upton, R., & Goldberg, A. (1997) *Botanical Safety Handbook* (p. 62). New York: CRC Press.

Ottariano, S. (1999). *Medicinal herbal therapy: A pharmacist's viewpoint* (pp. 132–134). North Hampton, NH: Nicolin Fields Publishing.

Werbach, M., & Murray, M. (1994). *Botanical influences on illness: A source book of clinical research* (pp. 23–24, 110, 203–204). CA: Third Line Press.

NOTES

NOTES

GOLDENSEAL
(Hydrastis canadensis)

Historical Uses

Sometimes called "poor man's ginseng," goldenseal was discovered by Cherokee Indians, who used it for eyewashes, acne, and eczema. The Food and Agriculture organization of the United Nations cites goldenseal as one of the best-selling herbs internationally. It is very bitter.

Growth

Goldenseal is found in wooded areas in eastern North America, but it is endangered because of overharvesting. The plant prefers moist soil and shade.

Part Used

• Root

Medical Uses

Goldenseal is used for infections of the mucous membranes, digestive disorders, gastritis, peptic ulcers, colitis, and traveler's diarrhea. It has been used to treat streptococcus, staphylococcus, and bacterial vaginosis. Goldenseal's major constituent (berberine) has also been effective in treating candidiasis (yeast infections). Scientists have disproved the rumor that goldenseal masks morphine in urine testing.

Dosage

Use standardized extract of 5 to 15 percent berberine.

Capsules: 250 to 500 mg three times a day. Combination products that contain goldenseal should be taken four times a day. Use goldenseal for only 1 week because it disrupts intestinal flora. A dose of *Lactobacillus acidophilus* should be given with goldenseal because it is a helpful bacteria for the intestine.

Warnings

• Goldenseal may interfere with vitamin B metabolism and may lower blood sugar levels. Experiments with animals suggest that it may cause nausea, vomiting, diarrhea, and slowing of breathing and heart rate at high doses.
• Don't take goldenseal if you are pregnant because it stimulates the uterus.
• Don't take goldenseal while breast-feeding.

This information is not intended to be a substitute for qualified medical intervention, counseling, or testing. Talk with your health-care practitioner if you are taking or considering taking any herbal medicine, especially if you are already taking prescription medications. If you experience ANY side effects, stop the herb and report the side effects to your health-care practitioner immediately.

GRAPE SEED

(Vitis vinifera)

Historical Uses

Grapes have been eaten and consumed in wines for centuries. Grape seed extract was patented in 1970 (McCaleb et al., 2000).

Growth

Wild grapes grow in warm regions of the northern hemisphere, South Africa, and South America.

Part Used

• Seed (red grape, crushed)

Major Chemical Compounds

• Essential fatty acids
• Vitamin E
• Procyanidins (antioxidant chemicals)
• Flavonoids

Clinical Uses

Grape seed extract is used as an antioxidant and for circulatory problems, varicose veins, sports injuries, and vision problems (McCaleb et al., 2000). It may be beneficial in the treatment of chronic pancreatitis (Bannerjee & Bagchi, 2001).

Mechanism of Action

Grape seed extract protects against free radicals, which results in its antioxidant effects. Procyanidins strengthen blood vessels. A beneficial effect of grape seed proanthocyanidins is the chemoprevention of cellular damage, although its mechanism is not clearly understood (Joshi et al., 2001).

Dosage

Grape seed extract is standardized to 85 to 95 percent procyanidins (McCaleb et al., 2000).

Capsules and tablets: 50 to 100 mg a day for prevention and 150 to 300 mg a day for illness (McCaleb, 2000; Bratman, 2000). May take up to 300 mg daily for a maximum of 3 weeks and then decrease to 40 to 80 mg for prevention (*Natural Medicines*, 2000). Always start with the lowest possible dose.

Side Effects

Grape seed extract may cause mild stomach upset, dizziness, and rash (McCaleb et al., 2000).

Contraindications

• None are known.

Herb-Drug Interactions

Large doses of grape seed should be used cautiously if the patient is taking an anticoagulant (Bratman, 2000).

Pregnancy and Breast-Feeding

No restrictions are known.

 # SUMMARY OF STUDIES

No recent clinical studies in humans are available.

REFERENCES

Bannerjee, B., & Bagchi, D. (2001). Beneficial effects of a novel ih636 grape seed proanthocyanidin extract in the treatment of chronic pancreatitis. *Digestion, 63*(3), 203–206.

Bratman, S., & Kroll, D. (2000). *The natural pharmacist: Your complete guide to illnesses and their natural remedies* (pp. 141–142). CA: Prima Publishing.

Joshi, S. S., Kuszynski, C. A., & Bagchi, D. (2001). The cellular and molecular basis of health benefits of grape seed proanthocyanidin extract. *Current Pharmaceutical Biotechnology, 2*(2), 187–200.

McCaleb, R., Leigh, E., & Morien, K. (2000). *The Encyclopedia of Popular Herbs.* Roseville, CA: Prima Publishing.

Natural Medicines Comprehensive Database. (2000). *Pharmacist's Letter and Prescriber's Letter.* Therapeutic Research Faculty.

NOTES

NOTES

GRAPE SEED
(Vitis vinifera)

Historical Uses

Grapes have been eaten and consumed in wines for centuries. Grape seed extract was patented in 1970 (McCaleb et al., 2000).

Growth

Wild grapes grow in warm regions of the northern hemisphere, South Africa, and South America.

Part Used

• Seed, red grape, crushed

Medical Uses

Grape seed extract is used as an antioxidant and for circulatory problems, varicose veins, sports injuries, and vision problems.

Dosage

Grape seed extract is standardized to 85 to 95 percent procyanidins.

Capsules and tablets: 50 to 100 mg a day for prevention and 150 to 300 mg a day for illness. May take up to 300 mg daily for a maximum of 3 weeks and then decrease to 40 to 80 mg for prevention. Always start with the lowest possible dose.

Warnings

• Grape seed may cause mild stomach upset, dizziness, and rash.
• Use grape seed cautiously if you take a blood thinner.

GREEN TEA
(Camellia sinensis)

Historical Uses

Green tea was first used by Buddhists in China and India and during meditation ceremonies in Japan. Traditional Chinese medicine recommends green tea "to prolong life" (Ferrara et al., 2001).

Growth

This herb comes from a small, native Chinese evergreen tree with green pointy leaves. It is grown primarily in China, India, and Japan.

Part Used

• Fresh leaves

Green tea comes from the fresh leaf, lightly steamed to avoid oxidation of the polyphenol components, in contrast to black tea,which is allowed to oxidize.

Major Chemical Compounds

• Polyphenols 8 to 12 percent
• Flavonoids (such as epigallo catechin gallate)
• Tannins
• Quercetin
• Alkaloids (such as caffeine)

Clinical Uses

Green tea is used as an antioxidant, for its anticancer effects, and for its effects as a sunscreen protection.

Mechanism of Action

Catechins have an antioxidant role in the prevention of certain cancers (Anderson et al., 2001). Polyphenols have antimutagenic and anticarcinogenic effects (Mukhatar et al., 1992; Stich, 1992; Katiyar et al., 1992; Wang et al., 1989; Richelle et al., 2001).

152

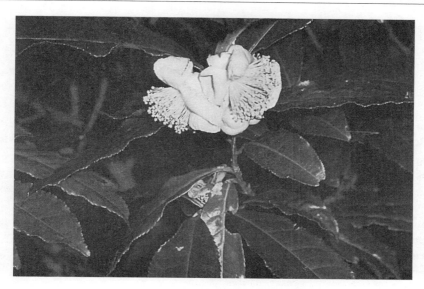

Dosage

Normal consumption in Japan is 3 cups per day with meals. Use 1 teaspoon of green tea leaves per cup of boiling water. Cool water slightly before steeping. Steep for about 3 minutes, strain, and drink. Antioxidants are released immediately in the cup. Do not reuse tea bags. Standardized green tea extract is 90 percent total polyphenols.

Side Effects

Green tea may elevate the international normalized ratio. It has milder caffeine side effects than black tea or coffee. Green tea made from tea bags contains about 29 to 47 mg of caffeine (1–5-minute brewing time); made from loose tea, it contains about 36 mg. Japanese green tea contains about 21 mg. Black tea made from loose tea has about 41 mg. Coffee made in a drip system has about 139 mg.

Contraindications

• Green tea is contraindicated for infants.

Herb-Drug Interactions

Green tea should be used cautiously if the patient is taking an anticoagulant.

Pregnancy and Breast-Feeding

Pregnant women should avoid caffeine.

Pediatric Patients

Green tea is not recommended for infants (McCaleb et al., 2000).

 SUMMARY OF STUDIES

Imai & Nakachi (March 1995). This cross-sectional study included 1371 men over age 40. Results: Green tea acted protectively against cardiovascular disease and disorders of the liver.

Stich (1992). This in vitro study suggests that taking green tea with food exerts a protective, beneficial effect.

Mukhatar et al. (1992). Data from this study suggest that polyphenols possess antimutagenic and anticarcinogenic effects.

Katiyar et al. (1992). This study found that green tea and its compounds could prevent carcinogenesis in animal tumor bioassay systems.

Wang et al. (1989). According to this study, green tea polyphenols affect carcinogen metabolism, DNA formation, and the scavenging of free radicals.

REFERENCES

Anderson, R. F., Fisher, L. J., Hara, Y., Harris, T., Mak, W. B., Medlton, L. D., & Packer, J. E. (2001). Green tea catechins partially protect DNA from (.)OH radical-induced strand breaks and base damage through fast chemical repair of DNA radicals. *Carcinogenesis, 22*(8), 1189–1193.

Ferrara, L., Montesano, D., & Senatore, A. (2001). The distribution of minerals and flavonoids in the tea plant (*Camellia sinensis*). *Farmaco, 56*(5–7), 397401.

Imai, K., & Nakachi, K. (1995). Cross sectional study of effects of drinking green tea on cardiovascular and liver diseases. *British Medical Journal, 310,* 693–696.

Katiyar, S., Agarwal, R., & Mukhatar, H. (1992). Green tea in chemoprevention of cancer. *Comprehensive Therapy, 18*(10), 3–8.

McCaleb, R., Leigh, E., & Morien, K. (2000). *The Encyclopedia of Popular Herbs.* Roseville, CA: Prima Publishing.

Mukhatar, H., Wang, Z., & Katiyar, S. (1992). Tea components: Antimutagenic and anticarcinogenic effects. *Preventive Medicine, 21,* 351–360.

Richelle, M., Tavazzi, I., & Offord, E. (2001). Comparison of the antioxidant activity of commonly consumed polyphenolic beverages (coffee, cocoa, and tea) prepared per cup serving. *Journal of Agriculture and Food Chemistry, 49*

Rosso, J. (1993). *Great good food* (p. 55). New York: Crown.

Stich, H. (1992). Teas and tea components as inhibitors of carcinogen formation in model systems and man. *Preventive Medicine, 21,* 377–384.

Wang, Z., Cheng, S., & Zhou, C. Antimutagenic activity of green tea polyphenols. *Mutation Research, 223,* 273–289.

NOTES

NOTES

GREEN TEA
(Camellia sinensis)

Historical Uses

Green tea was first used by Buddhists in China and India and during meditation ceremonies in Japan.

Growth

This herb comes from a small, native Chinese evergreen tree with green pointy leaves. It is grown primarily in China, India, and Japan.

Part Used

• Fresh leaf

Green tea comes from the fresh leaf, lightly steamed to avoid oxidation of the polyphenol components, in contrast to black tea, which is allowed to oxidize.

Medical Uses

Green tea is used as an antioxidant, for its anticancer effects, and for its effects as a sunscreen protection.

Dosage

Normal consumption in Japan is 3 cups per day with meals. Use 1 teaspoon of green tea leaves per cup of boiling water; cool water slightly before steeping. Steep for about 3 minutes, strain and drink. Antioxidants are released immediately in the cup. Do not reuse tea bags. Standardized green tea extract is 90 percent total polyphenols.

Warnings

• Green tea has milder caffeine side effects than black tea or coffee. Green tea made from tea bags contains about 29 to 47 mg of caffeine (1–5-minute brewing time); made from loose tea, it contains about 36 mg. Japanese green tea contains about 21 mg. Black tea made from loose tea has about 41 mg. Coffee made in a drip system has about 139 mg.
• Green tea should not be given to infants.
• Use green tea cautiously if you take a blood thinner. Green tea may increase the risk of bleeding.
• Pregnant women should avoid caffeine.

HAWTHORN
(Crataegus oxyacantha, Crataegus laevigata)

Historical Uses

Hawthorn was the symbol of hope and happiness in ancient Greece and Rome.

Growth

This shrub grows in temperate zones in Europe and in the United States.

Parts Used

- Berries
- Flower heads
- Leaves

Major Chemical Compounds

- Flavonoids
- Oligomeric procyanidins
- Cardiotonic amines
- Anthocyanins

Clinical Uses

Hawthorn is used as a heart tonic and for high blood pressure, high cholesterol, and angina.

Mechanism of Action

Flavonoids prevent destruction of collagen, prevent plaque buildup, and strengthen blood vessels (Murray, 1995). Inotropic in nature, they help the heart muscle to contract. Anthocyanins inhibit low-density lipoprotein oxidation and platelet aggregation, which protects against heart disease. They help to treat vascular disorders and also capillary fragility (Craig, 1999). Flavonoids cause smooth muscles of coronary vessels to dilate, increasing blood flow and decreasing angina (Tyler, 1994). Proanthocyanidins in the flower heads inhibit biosynthesis of thromboxane A2 (Vibes et al., 1994).

Dosage

Hawthorn extracts are standardized to 2.2 percent flavonoids or 18 percent oligomeric procyanidins (McCaleb, et al., 2000).

Capsules: Starting dose is 80 mg twice daily, increased to 960 mg daily (Ottariano, 1999).

Tincture (1:5): 5 mL three times daily (McCaleb et al., 2000).

Tea: 1 to 2 teaspoons of hawthorn berries in 250 mL of water, steeped for 15 minutes (McCaleb et al., 2000).

Side Effects

None are known (McGuffin et al., 1997).

Contraindications

• None are known.

Herb-Drug Interactions

Hawthorn may enhance the effects of cardiac glycosides (McGuffin et al., 1997) and may interact with theophylline, caffeine, papaverine, sodium nitrate, adenosine, epinephrine, and barbiturates (Blumenthal, 2000). It also may interfere with or intensify the effects of digoxin.

Pregnancy and Breast-Feeding

No restrictions are known. (McGuffin et al., 1997). However, Ottariano (1999) and *Natural Medicines* (2000) do not recommend the use of hawthorn during pregnancy and lactation.

SUMMARY OF STUDIES

Hanak & Bruckel (1983). This double-blind, placebo-controlled study lasted 3 weeks and included 60 subjects with angina pectoris who took 180 mg/day of hawthorn extract, divided into three doses. Results: Pathological ECG changes caused by exertion improved significantly in treated versus control subjects and caused no side effects.

Schmidt et al. (1994). Seventy-eight patients with chronic heart disease were given 600 mg/day of hawthorn extract. Results: Subjects who took hawthorn had decreased blood pressure, decreased heart rate, and decreased shortness of breath while exercising compared to subjects who did not take hawthorn.

REFERENCES

Blumenthal, M. (2000). Interactions between herbs and conventional drugs: Introductory considerations. *HerbalGram, 49,* 52–63.

Craig, W. J. (1999). Health-promoting properties of common herbs. *American Journal of Clinical Nutrition, 70*(3), 491S–499S.

159

Hanak, T., & Bruckel, M. (1983). Treatment of moderately stable forms of angina pectoris with *Crataegutt novo* [in German]. *Therapiewoche, 33,* 4331–4333.

McCaleb, R., Leigh, E., & Morien, K. (2000). *The Encyclopedia of Popular Herbs.* Roseville, CA: Prima Publishing.

McGuffin, M., Hobbs, C., Upton, R., & Goldberg, A. (1997) *Botanical Safety Handbook.* New York: CRC.

Murray, M. (1995). *The Healing Power of Herbs.* Roseville, CA: Prima Publishing.

Natural Medicines Comprehensive Database (pp. 543–547) (2000). *Pharmacist's Letter and Prescriber's Letter.* Therapeutic Research Faculty.

Ottariano, S. (1999). *Medicinal herbal therapy: A pharmacist's viewpoint* (pp. 138–141). North Hampton, NH: Nicolin Fields Publishing.

Schmidt, U., Kuhn, U., Ploch, M., et al. (1994). Efficacy of the Hawthorne (*Crataegus*) preparation LI 132 in 78 patients with chronic CHF defined as NYHA functional class II. *Phytomedicine, 1:*17–24.

Tyler, V. (1994). *Herbs of choice.* Binghamton, NY: Pharmaceutical Products Press.

Vibes, J., Lasserre, B., Gleye, J., & Declume, C. (1994). Inhibition of thromboxane A2 biosynthesis in vitro by the main components of Crataegus oxyacanthan (Hawthorne) flower heads. *Prostaglandins Leukot Essential Fatty Acids* 50:173–175 [Medline].

NOTES

HAWTHORN
(Crataegus oxyacantha, Crataegus laevigata)

Historical Uses

Hawthorn was the symbol of hope and happiness in ancient Greece and Rome.

Growth

This shrub grows in temperate zones in Europe and the United States.

Parts Used

- Berries
- Flower heads
- Leaves

Medical Uses

Hawthorn is used as a heart tonic and for high blood pressure, high cholesterol, and angina.

Dosage

Hawthorn extracts are standardized to 2.2 percent flavonoids or 18 percent oligomeric procyanidins.

Capsules: Start with 80 mg twice daily, increasing to 960 mg daily.

Tincture (1:5): 5 mL three times daily.

Tea: 1 to 2 teaspoons of hawthorn berries in 250 mL of water, steeped for 15 minutes.

Warnings

- No side effects or contraindications are known.
- Don't use hawthorn if you take any of the following medications: heart medications (such as digoxin), theophylline, caffeine, papaverine, sodium nitrate, adenosine, epinephrine, or a barbiturate.
- Don't use hawthorn if you are pregnant or breast-feeding. Consult your health-care practitioner.

HOREHOUND, WHITE

(Marrubium vulgare)

Historical Uses

In folk medicine, horehound has been used primarily for expelling worms; stimulating menses; and treating cough (horehound drops), dog bites, and fevers. In Egypt, horehound was known as "Eye of the Star" (Weiss & Weiss, 1985).

Growth

A member of the mint family, horehound has hairy leaves and stems. It grows in the United States and Europe and likes sandy soil, warmth, and sun. It can be planted by seed or cuttings (Weiss & Weiss, 1985). Harvest horehound leaves to about 4 inches above the ground before flowering (Weiss & Weiss, 1985).

Parts Used

- Dried leaves
- Flowering tops

Major Chemical Compounds

- Marrubin
- Bitters
- Mucilage
- Tannins

Clinical Uses

Traditional use has been for bronchitis and respiratory illness with a nonproductive cough. Horehound also may have a hypoglycemic effect (Roman Ramos et al., 1992). It has been approved by the German Commission E for "loss of appetite, bloating and flatulence" (Blumenthal et al., 2000).

Mechanism of Action

This herb's bitterness aids digestion. It also exerts expectorant, antispasmodic, and antinociceptive (decreasing painful stimuli) effects by an unknown mechanism, but it is not known if horehound does not interact with opioid systems and is not reversed by naloxone (DeJesus et al., 2000).

Dosage

Tea: Pour 150 mL of boiling water over 1 to 2 grams of finely cut leaves and steep for 5 to 10 minutes. Then strain and drink up to three times a day (*Natural Medicines*, 2000).

Lozenges: Use as needed.

Side Effects

Horehound may lower blood glucose levels. Large doses may induce cardiac irregularities.

Contraindications

• Horehound is contraindicated during pregnancy.

Herb-Drug Interactions

Use cautiously in diabetic patients who take insulin or other antidiabetic agents (Roman Ramos et al., 1992).

Pregnancy and Breast-Feeding

Do not use horehound in pregnant patients because it is an abortifacient (induces abortion) (Brinker, 1998) and because it stimulates the uterus and menstrual flow (McGuffin et al., 1997). No restrictions are known for breast-feeding patients (McGuffin et al., 1997).

 SUMMARY OF STUDIES

No recent clinical studies in humans are available.

REFERENCES

Blumenthal, M., Goldberg, A., & Brinckmann, J. (Eds.). (2000). *Herbal medicine expanded Commission E monographs.* Austin, TX: American Botanical Council; Newton, MA: Integrative Medicine Communications.

Brinker, F. (1998). *Herb contraindications and drug interactions.* (2nd ed.). Sandy, Oregon: Eclectic Medical Publications.

DeJesus, R., et al. (2000). Analysis of the antinociceptive properties of marrubiin isolated from *Marrubiim vulgare. Phytomedicine, 7*(2), 111–115.

McGuffin, M., Hobbs, C., Upton, R., & Goldberg, A. (1997) *Botanical Safety Handbook.* New York: CRC.

Natural Medicines Comprehensive Database. (2000). *Pharmacist's Letter and Prescriber's Letter.* Therapeutic Research Faculty.

Roman Ramos, R., Alarcon-Aguilar, F., Lara-Lemus, A., & Flores-Saenz, J. (1992, Spring). Hypoglycemic effect of plants used in Mexico as antidiabetics. *Archives of Medical Research, 23*(1), 59–64.

Weiss, G., & Weiss, S. (1985). *Growing and using the healing herbs*. Emmaus, PA: Rodale Press.

NOTES

HOREHOUND, WHITE
(Marrubium vulgare)

Historical Uses

In folk medicine, horehound has been used primarily for expelling worms, stimulating menses, and treating cough (horehound drops), dog bites, and fevers. In Egypt, horehound was known as "Eye of the Star."

Growth

A member of the mint family, horehound has hairy leaves and stems. It grows in the United States and Europe and likes sandy soil, warmth, and sun. It can be planted by seed or cuttings. Harvest horehound leaves to about 4 inches above the ground before flowering.

Parts Used

- Dried leaves
- Flowering tops

Medical Uses

Traditional use has been for bronchitis and respiratory illness with a nonproductive cough. Horehound also has been shown to lower blood sugar levels.

Dosage

Tea: Pour 150 mL of boiling water over 1 to 2 grams of finely cut leaves and steep for 5 to 10 minutes. Then strain and drink up to three times a day.

Lozenges: Use as needed.

Warnings

- Horehound may lower blood sugar levels.
- Large doses of horehound may cause changes in heart rate.
- Don't use horehound if you take insulin or another antidiabetic medication.
- Don't use horehound if you are pregnant because it stimulates the uterus, promotes menstrual flow, and may induce abortion.
- No restrictions are known during breast-feeding.

RECIPES

HOMEMADE HOREHOUND COUGH SYRUP

Pick a few fresh horehound leaves and chop them finely. Add 1½ teaspoons of chopped leaves to 8 ounces of water and steep for 10 minutes. Then strain the herb and add twice as much honey to the liquid. Mix and take 1 teaspoon four times daily for coughs.

HORSE CHESTNUT
(Aesculus hippocastanum)

Historical Uses

Historically, horse chestnut seeds were used as an anticoagulant and for nocturnal leg cramps (McCaleb et al., 2000).

Growth

The deciduous horse chestnut tree grows in the northern hemisphere. It prefers well-drained soil and sun or partial shade.

Part Used

- Seed extract

Major Chemical Compounds

- Triterpenic saponin aescin

Clinical Uses

Horse chestnut is used to improve circulation and to treat leg cramps, varicose veins, hemorrhoids, and chronic venous insufficiency (Diehm et al., 1996). It is approved by the German Commission E for "chronic venous insufficiency" (Blumenthal et al., 2000).

Mechanism of Action

Horse chestnut has anti-inflammatory effects (Calabrese & Preston, 1993). It also reduces capillary permeability, protects the integrity of the veins, and reduces levels of leukocytes and proteoglycan hydrolases in limbs affected by chronic venous insufficiency.

Dosage

Seed extract: 300 mg twice daily, standardized to contain 15 to 21 percent aescin. Some studies used 50 mg of aescin per capsule twice a day (Diehm et al., 1996). Do not make tea out of raw, unprocessed horse chestnut seeds (McCaleb et al., 2000).

Gel or lotion: Apply 2 percent aescin gel or lotion topically four times a day to bruises, strains, sprains, and varicose veins.

Side Effects

Horse chestnut may cause nausea, stomach complaints, and itching (Blumenthal et al., 2000).

Contraindications

- Do not use horse chestnut with anticoagulants (McCaleb et al., 2000) or if patient has kidney or liver disease.
- Do not apply gel to broken skin.
- Do not make tea out of raw, unprocessed horse chestnut seeds (McCaleb et al., 2000).

Herb-Drug Interactions

None are known.

Pregnancy and Breast-Feeding

Avoid use in pregnant and breast-feeding women (Bown, 1995).

SUMMARY OF STUDIES

Calabrese & Preston (1993). This study is a double-blind, randomized, single-dose trial of topical 2 percent aescin gel in subjects with hematomas. Results: Bruises healed more quickly in subjects who had horse chestnut applied topically compared with those who received placebo.

Pittler & Ernst (1998). This is a meta-analysis of 13 studies. Results: Horse chestnut was superior to placebo in improving symptoms of chronic venous insufficiency.

REFERENCES

Blumenthal, M., Goldberg, A., & Brinckmann, J. (Eds.). (2000). *Herbal medicine expanded Commission E monographs.* Austin, TX: American Botanical Council; Newton, MA: Integrative Medicine Communications.

Bown, D. (1995). *The Herb Society of America encyclopedia of herbs and their uses.* New York: Dorling Kindersley Publishing.

Calabrese, C., & Preston, P.(1993). Reports of a double-blind, randomized, single-dose trial of a topical 2% escin gel versus placebo in the acute treatment of experimentally induced hematoma in volunteers. *Planta Medica, 59,* 394–397.

Diehm, C., Trampisch, J., Lange, S., & Schmidt, C. (1996). Comparison of leg compression stocking and oral horse-chestnut seed extract therapy in patients with chronic venous insufficiency. *The Lancet, 347,* 292–294.

McCaleb, R., Leigh, E., & Morien, K. (2000). *The Encyclopedia of Popular Herbs.* Roseville, CA: Prima Publishing.

Pittler, M. H, & Ernst, E.(1998). Horse chestnut seed extract for chronic venous insufficiency: a criteria-based systematic review. *Archives of Dermatology, 134,* 1356–1360.

NOTES

NOTES

HORSE CHESTNUT
(Aesculus hippocastanum)

Historical Uses

Historically, horse chestnut seeds were used as an anticoagulant and for nocturnal leg cramps.

Growth

The deciduous horse chestnut tree grows in the northern hemisphere. It prefers well-drained soil and sun or partial shade.

Part Used

• Seed extract

Medical Uses

Horse chestnut is used to improve circulation for varicose veins and to treat leg cramps and hemorrhoids.

Dosage

Seed extract: 300 mg twice daily, standardized to contain 15 to 21 percent aescin. Some studies used 50 mg of aescin per capsule twice a day. Don't make tea out of raw, unprocessed horse chestnut seeds.

Gel or lotion: Apply 2 percent aescin gel or lotion four times a day to bruises, strains, sprains, and varicose veins.

Warnings

• Horse chestnut may cause nausea, stomach complaints, or itching.
• Don't use horse chestnut if you take a blood thinner or if you have kidney or liver disease.
• Don't apply gel or lotion to broken skin.
• Don't make tea out of raw, unprocessed horse chestnut seeds.
• Avoid use during pregnancy and breast-feeding.

HORSERADISH
(Armoracia rusticana)

Historical Uses

In folklore, horseradish was used to treat urinary tract infections (UTIs) and respiratory congestion.

Growth

This perennial plant grows in Europe and North America. It prefers sun and well-drained soil. It is said to protect potatoes from Colorado beetles (Bown, 1995).

Part Used

- Root

Major Chemical Compounds

- Mustard oil
- Sinigrin
- Iron
- Potassium

Clinical Uses

Horseradish is approved by the German Commission E for "catarrhs of the respiratory tract and supportive therapy for UTIs" (Blumenthal et al., 2000).

Mechanism of Action

Horseradish has stimulant and diuretic effects (Hoffman, 1992).

Dosage

Root: Can be grated in small amounts and up to 20 grams a day added to food.

Tea: Pour 1 cup of boiling water over 1 teaspoon of chopped herb, infuse for 5 minutes, and drink three times a day or more often to help flu symptoms (Hoffman, 1992).

Poultice: Apply externally as a poultice (grate horseradish, wrap in a cloth, and place on chest) to ease congestion in bronchitis.

Side Effects

Horseradish may cause stomach distress if used in large amounts.

Contraindications

- Horseradish is not recommended for patients with stomach or duodenal ulcers (Blumenthal et al., 2000; McGuffin et al., 1997).
- It is not recommended for patients with hypothyroid conditions (*Natural Medicines*, 2000).

Herb-Drug Interactions

Horseradish may interfere with levothyroxine or hypothyroid condition (*Natural Medicines*, 2000).

Pregnancy and Breast-Feeding

Horseradish is not recommended for pregnant or breast-feeding patients (Blumenthal et al., 2000).

Pediatric Patients

Horseradish is not recommended for children under age 4 (Blumenthal et al., 2000).

SUMMARY OF STUDIES

No recent clinical studies in humans are available.

REFERENCES

Blumenthal, M., Goldberg, A., & Brinckmann, J. (Eds.). (2000). *Herbal medicine expanded Commission E monographs.* Austin, TX: American Botanical Council; Newton, MA: Integrative Medicine Communications.

Blumenthal, M., Busse, W., Goldberg, A., Gruenwald, J., Hall, T., Riggins, C., & Rister, R. (Eds.). (1998). *The complete German Commission E monographs: Therapeutic guide to herbal medicines.* (S. Klein & R. Rister, Trans.). Austin, TX: American Botanical Council; Newton, MA: Integrative Medicine Communications.

Bown, D. (1995). *The Herb Society of America encyclopedia of herbs and their uses* (p. 242). New York: Dorling Kindersley Publishing.

Chichon, P. (August, 2000). Herbs and the common cold. *Advance for Nurse Practitioners.*

Hoffman, D. (1992). *The new holistic herbal* (p. 207). Boston: Element Books Limited.

McGuffin, M., Hobbs, C., Upton, R., & Goldberg, A. (1997). *Botanical safety handbook* (p. 14). Boca Raton, FL: CRC Press.

Natural Medicines Comprehensive Database. (2000). *Pharmacist's Letter and Prescriber's Letter* (pp. 574–575). Therapeutic Research Faculty.

NOTES

HORSERADISH
(Armoracia rusticana)

Historical Uses

In folklore, horseradish was used to treat urinary tracts infections and respiratory congestion.

Growth

This perennial plant grows in Europe and North America. It prefers sun and well-drained soil. It is said to protect potatoes from Colorado beetles.

Part Used

• Root

Medical Uses

Horseradish is used to treat urinary tract infections and respiratory congestion. A pungent herb, it helps you to perspire. Horseradish is high in iron and potassium.

Dosage

Root: Can be grated in small amounts and up to 20 grams a day added to food.

Leaves: May be added to salads.

Tea: Pour 1 cup of boiling water over 1 teaspoon of chopped herb, infuse for 5 minutes, and drink three times a day or more often to help flu symptoms.

Poultice: Apply externally as a poultice (grate horseradish, wrap in a cloth, and place on chest) to ease congestion in bronchitis.

Warnings

• Horseradish may cause stomach distress if used in large amounts.
• It is not recommended for patients with stomach or duodenal ulcers or thyroid disease.
• Don't use horseradish if you take levothyroxine or other thyroid medications.
• Don't use horseradish if you are pregnant or breast-feeding.
• Don't give horseradish to children under age 4.
• Cooking destroys the volatile oils that help to give horseradish its medicinal effects.

RECIPES

A ZESTY CONDIMENT

Mix grated horseradish with sour cream and use as a condiment on beef.

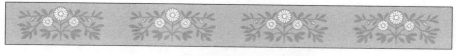

HYSSOP
(Hyssopus officinalis)

Historical Use

Hyssop, which is Greek for "holy herb," was used to cleanse and purify for sacredness.

Growth

This perennial shrub of the Lamiaceae family grows on the sides of roads and can be planted in herb gardens. The leaves and flowers have a camphorlike odor and a bitter taste because of their volatile oils (Tyler, 1993). Hyssop can be planted next to cabbage plants to deter insects.

Parts Used

• Dried aerial (above-ground) parts

Major Chemical Compounds

• Terpenoids
• Volatile acids
• Flavonoids
• Lyssopin
• Tannin

Clinical Uses

Hyssop is used for asthma, bronchitis, and coughs and as an expectorant, a diaphoretic, and a stimulant.

Mechanism of Action

Caffeic acid, unidentified tannins, and unidentified higher molecular weight compounds exhibit strong anti-HIV activity, which may be useful in treating patients with AIDS (Kreis et al., 1990; Gollapudi et al., 1995).

Dosage

Tea as an infusion: Steep 1 to 2 teaspoon of dried flower tops in 150 mL of boiling water for 10 to 15 minutes. Strain and drink up to three times a day (Natural Medicines, 2000; Hoffman, 1992).

Gargle: Tea may be used as a gargle (*Natural Medicines, 2000*).

Tincture: 1 to 4 mL three times a day (Hoffman, 1992).

Side Effects

Hyssop may promote menstruation and stimulate the uterus. Seizures have been reported in two adults and one child using essential oil of hyssop (Burkhard et al., 1999).

Contraindications

• Hyssop is contraindicated in pregnant patients.

Herb-Drug Interactions

None are known.

Pregnancy and Breast-Feeding

Avoid use in pregnant and breast-feeding patients because the herb stimulates the uterus and menstruation (McGuffin et al., 1997).

SUMMARY OF STUDIES

No recent clinical studies in humans are available.

REFERENCES

Bown, D. (1995). *The Herb Society of America encyclopedia of herbs and their uses.* New York: Dorling Kindersley Publishing.

Burkhard, P., Burkhardt, K., Haenggeli, C., & Landis, T. (1999). Plant-induced seizures: reappearance of an old problem. *Journal of Neurology, 246*(8), 667–670.

Gollapudi, S., Sharma, H. A., Aggarwal, S., Byers, L. D., Ensley, H. E., & Gupta, S. (1995). Isolation of a previously unidentified polysaccharide (MAR 10) from *Hyssop officinalis* that exhibits strong activity against human immunodeficiency virus type 1. *Biochemical and Biophysical Research Communications, 210*(1), 145–151.

Hoffman, D. (1992). *The new holistic herbal.* Boston: Element Books Limited.

Kreus, W., et al. (1990). Inhibition of HIV replication by *Hyssop officinalis* extracts. *Antiviral Research, 14*(6), 323–337.

McGuffin, M., Hobbs, C., Upton, R., & Goldberg, A. (1997) *Botanical Safety Handbook* (p. 63). New York: CRC.

Natural Medicines Comprehensive Database. (2000). *Pharmacist's Letter and Prescriber's Letter* (pp. 583–584). Therapeutic Research Faculty.

Tyler, V. (1993). *The honest herbal* (pp. 183–184). Binghamton, NY: Pharmaceutical Products Press.

NOTES

NOTES

HYSSOP
(Hyssopus officinalis)

Historical Use

Hyssop, which is Greek for "holy herb," was used to cleanse and purify for sacredness.

Growth

This perennial shrub of the Lamiaceae family grows on the sides of roads and can be planted in herb gardens. The leaves and flowers have a camphorlike odor and a bitter taste because of their volatile oils. Plant hyssop next to cabbage plants to deter insects.

Parts Used

• Dried aerial (above-ground) parts

Medical Uses

Hyssop is used for asthma, bronchitis, and coughs and as an expectorant, a diaphoretic, and a stimulant.

Dosage

Tea as an infusion: Steep 1 to 2 teaspoon of dried flower tops in 150 mL of boiling water for 10 to 15 minutes. Strain and drink up to three times a day.

Gargle: Tea may be used as a gargle.

Tincture: 1 to 4 mL three times a day.

Leaves: Hyssop leaves have a bitter, sage-mint flavor and may complement legumes and meat dishes.

Warnings

• Don't use hyssop if you are pregnant; it may stimulate the uterus and promote menstruation.
• Seizures have been reported in two adults and one child using essential oil of hyssop.
• Avoid use while breast-feeding.

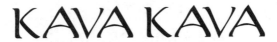

KAVA KAVA
(Piper methysticum)

Historical Uses

Kava comes from a Greek word meaning "intoxicating." The herb has been used in Polynesian countries to make a ceremonial drink.

Growth

This tropical, perennial shrub is a member of the pepper family and is native to Oceania.

Part Used

• Root

Major Chemical Compound

• Kavalactones

Clinical Uses

Kava kava is used to improve mental function and for nonpsychotic anxiety disorders, hot flashes, and anxiety and mild depression associated with menopause (De Leo et al., 2000; Morien, 1998). It is approved by the German Commission E for "anxiety, stress, and restlessness" (Blumenthal et al., 2000).

Mechanism of Action

Kava kava has sedative, analgesic, anticonvulsant, and muscle relaxant effects and acts on the limbic system. Its action is different from that of aspirin, morphine, and benzodiazepines. Little information is currently available on kavalactones (Dentali, 1997).

For anxiety:

Standardized extract: 70 mg kavalactones two to three times daily (McCaleb et al., 2000).

Capsules or tablets: 400 to 500 mg up to six times daily.

Tincture (1:2): 15 to 30 drops up to three times daily (Foster, 1998). Tincture drops may be added to a small amount of water or juice. Recommended use up to 3 months (McGuffin et al., 1997). Total kavalactones should not exceed 300 mg per day (McGuffin, 2000).

Tea: Does not extract important kavalactones.

Side Effects

Side effects are rare. They include liver damage, yellowing of the skin with chronic abuse, and depression of the nervous system.

Contraindications

- Kava kava is contraindicated in patients who have depression of biological origin (Blumenthal et al., 2000).
- Do not give kava kava to a patient who will be driving or operating heavy machinery (McGuffin, 2000). In one reported case, a man who drank more than 8 cups of kava kava was charged with driving under the influence.
- This herb is contraindicated in children under age 18 (McGuffin, 2000).

Herb-Drug Interactions

Kava kava may potentiate the effects of alcohol and other central nervous system depressants (Blumenthal, 2000). Additive effects have been noted with alprazolam. The efficacy of levodopa may be reduced by kava kava (Blumenthal, 2000).

Pregnancy and Breast-Feeding

Avoid use in pregnant or breast-feeding women (McGuffin et al., 1997).

 # SUMMARY OF STUDIES

Volz & Kieser (1997). This double-blind, 25-week trial included 101 men and women who were diagnosed with at least one of five anxiety disorders. Standardized kava kava extract (WS 1490) was compared to placebo. Results: The long-term efficacy of kava kava was superior to that of placebo. Two patients reported stomach upset.

Woelk et al. (1993). This double-blind, 6-week comparative study included 164 patients with nonpsychotic anxiety. They took kava kava extract 210 mg, oxazepam 15 mg, or bromezepam 9 mg. Results: Kava kava did as well in reducing anxiety as the two benzodiazepine-type anxiolytic drugs.

De Leo et al. (2000). In a randomized controlled trial, 40 menopausal women were given hormone replacement therapy (HRT) and kava kava or HRT and placebo. Significant reductions in anxiety were noted at 3 and 6 months in the HRT and kava kava group.

Pittler and Ernst (2000). In a review of the literature and meta-analysis, studies concluded that kava kava extract was superior to placebo in treating the symptoms of anxiety.

REFERENCES

Blumenthal, M. (2000). Interactions between herbs and conventional drugs: Introductory considerations. *HerbalGram, 49,* 52–63.

Blumenthal, M., Goldberg, A., & Brinckmann, J. (Eds.). (2000). *Herbal medicine expanded Commission E monographs* (pp. 221–225). Austin, TX: American Botanical Council; Newton, MA: Integrative Medicine Communications.

De Leo, V., La Marca, A., Lanzetta, D., Palazzi, S., Torricelli, M., Facchini, C., & Morgante, G. (2000). Assessment of the association of kava-kava extract and hormone replacement therapy in the treatment of postmenopause anxiety [in Italian]. *Minerva Ginecologica (Torino), 52*(6), 263–267.

Dentali, S. (1997). HRF produces safety review on kava for AHPA. *HerbalGram, 40,* 14.

Foster, S. (1998). *101 medicinal herbs.* Loveland, CO: Interweave Press.

McCaleb, R., Leigh, E., & Morien, K. (2000). *The Encyclopedia of Popular Herbs* (pp. 273–275). Roseville, CA: Prima Publishing.

McGuffin, M. (2000). Self regulatory initiatives by the herbal industry. *HerbalGram, 48,* 42–43.

McGuffin, M., Hobbs, C., Upton, R., & Goldberg, A. (1997) *Botanical Safety Handbook* (p. 86). New York: CRC.

Morien, K. (1998, Summer). Kava (*Piper methysticum*). *Herb Research Foundation,* 4–5.

Pittler, M. H., & Ernst, E. (2000). Efficacy of kava extract for treating anxiety: Systematic review and meta-analysis. *Journal of Clinical Psychopharmacology, 20*(1), 84–89.

Volz, H. P., & Kieser, M. (1997). Kava-kava extract WS 1490 versus placebo in anxiety disorders—A randomized placebo-controlled 25-week outpatient trial. *Pharmacopsychiatry, 30,* 1–5.

NOTES

KAVA KAVA
(Piper methysticum)

Historical Uses

Kava comes from a Greek word meaning "intoxicating." The herb has been used in Polynesian countries to make a ceremonial drink.

Growth

This tropical, perennial shrub is a member of the pepper family and is native to Oceania.

Part Used

• Root

Medical Uses

Kava kava is used to improve mental function and for anxiety disorders, hot flashes, and anxiety and mild depression associated with menopause.

Dosage

For anxiety:

Standardized extract: 70 mg kavalactones two to three times daily.

Capsules or tablets: 400 to 500 mg up to six times daily.

Tincture (1:2): 15 to 30 drops up to three times daily. Tincture drops may be added to a small amount of water or juice. Recommended use up to 3 months. Total kavalactones should not exceed 300 mg per day.

Tea: Does not extract important chemical kavalactones.

Warnings

• Side effects are rare. They include liver damage, yellowing of the skin with chronic abuse, and depression of the nervous system.
• This herb should not be used by persons with certain types of depression. Discuss this with your health-care practitioner.
• Don't drive or operate heavy machinery when taking kava kava. In one reported case, a man who drank more than 8 cups of kava kava was charged with driving under the influence.
• Don't give kava kava to children under age 18.

- Don't take kava kava with alcohol or other central nervous system depressants, alprazolam, or levodopa (medication for Parkinson's disease).
- Don't take kava kava if you are pregnant or breast-feeding.

This information is not intended to be a substitute for qualified medical intervention, counseling, or testing. Talk with your health-care practitioner if you are taking or considering taking any herbal medicine, especially if you are already taking prescription medications. If you experience ANY side effects, stop the herb and report the side effects to your health-care practitioner immediately.

LEMON BALM
(Melissa officinalis)

Historical Uses

Paracelsus called lemon balm "the elixir of life" (Bown D, 1995). Benedictine missionaries first brought lemon balm to the West. Historically, leaves were picked fresh and used as a poultice to reduce inflammation and a cup of lemon balm tea was used to reduce a fever.

Melissa means "honeybee" in Greek. If smeared on hives, lemon balm will attract bees.

Growth

Lemon balm is a member of the Lamiaceae family and is native to southern Europe. The plant grows indoors or out, and it prefers moist soil with partial shade. The leaves are lemon scented.

Part Used

• Leaves

Major Chemical Compounds

• Citral
• Citonellal
• Geraniol
• Flavonoids
• Quercitin

Clinical Uses

Lemon balm is used as a sleep aid (Cerny et al., 1999) and for nervousness and stomachaches. It is used externally for oral herpes (Mohrig & Alken, 1996). In Europe, lemon balm topical cream is used to treat oral and genital herpes (Bratman & Kroll, 2000). It is approved by the German Commission E for "nervous sleeping disorders and gastrointestinal complaints" (Blumenthal et al., 2000).

Mechanism of Action

The actions of lemon balm are unknown. One theory is that lemon balm may make it difficult for the herpes virus to attach to cells (Bratman & Kroll, 2000).

Dosage

Tea: Pour one cup of boiling water over 1 to 2 teaspoons of finely chopped leaves and steep for 5 minutes.

Extract cream (external use): Apply standard *Melissa* 70:1 extract cream in a thick layer at the first sign of blisters four times a day up to 14 days. Also may be used on a regular basis twice a day to prevent oral herpes (Bratman & Kroll, 2000).

Side Effects

None are known.

Contraindications

• None are known.

Herb-Drug Interactions

None are known.

Pregnancy and Breast-Feeding

Lemon balm is safe if used at recommended dosages (McGuffin et al., 1997).

SUMMARY OF STUDIES

Mohrig & Alken (1996). This double-blind, placebo-controlled, randomized, two-armed clinical trial included 116 patients; 58 were treated topically with a highly concentrated and fractionated 70:1 extract of *Melissa* in a cream base (1 percent Melissa extract cream), and 58 were treated with a placebo in a cream base. Patients were treated for herpes simplex 2 to 4 times daily over 5 to 10 days or until the area was healed. Of the 116 patients, 67 had herpes labialis. Results: Statistical differences were seen on day 2 of the study among patients who used *Melissa* extract compared to those who used the placebo and with patients who started therapy within 4 hours of symptom onset.

Cerny et al. (1999). This double-blind, placebo-controlled, multicenter study included 88 healthy volunteers who did not have insomnia. Subjects took a valerian/lemon balm combination (Songha Night from Switzerland, containing 480 mg valerian dry extract [4.5:1] and 240 mg lemon balm dry extract [5:1]) 30 minutes before bedtime. Results: Improvement in sleep quality without serious side effects.

REFERENCES

Blumenthal, M., Goldberg, A., & Brinckmann, J. (Eds.). (2000). *Herbal medicine expanded Commission E monographs* (pp. 230–232). Austin, TX: American Botanical Council; Newton, MA: Integrative Medicine Communications.

Bown, D. (1995). *The Herb Society of America encyclopedia of herbs and their uses.* New York: Dorling Kindersley Publishing.

Bratman, S., & Kroll, D. (2000). *The natural pharmacist: Your complete guide to illnesses and their natural remedies* (pp. 141–142). CA: Prima Publishing.

Cerny, A., & Schmid, K. (1999). Tolerability and efficacy of valerian/lemon balm in healthy volunteers (a double-blind, placebo-controlled, multicentre study). *Filoterapia, 70,* 221–228.

McGuffin, M., Hobbs, C., Upton, R., & Goldberg, A. (1997) *Botanical Safety Handbook* (p. 75). New York: CRC.

Mohrig, A., & Alken, R. (1996). Meta-analysis of a placebo-controlled clinical trial of Lomaherpan treatment in Herpes simplex at various locations. Berlin.

Vogt, H., et al. (1988). Melissenextrakt bei Herpes simplex. *Der Allgemeinarzt, 13,* 3–151.

Wobling, R., & Leonhardt, K. (1994). Local therapy of Herpes simplex with dried extract from *Melissa officinalis. Phytomedicine, 1,* 25–31.

Wood, R. (1999). *The new whole foods encyclopedia* (p. 189). New York: Penguin Press.

NOTES

NOTES

LEMON BALM
(Melissa officinalis)

Historical Uses

Paracelsus called lemon balm "the elixir of life." Benedictine missionaries first brought lemon balm to the West. Historically, leaves were picked fresh and used as a poultice to reduce inflammation and a cup of lemon balm tea was used to reduce a fever.

Melissa means "honeybee" in Greek. If smeared on hives, lemon balm will attract bees.

Growth

Lemon balm is a member of the Lamiaceae family and is native to southern Europe. The plant grows indoors or out, and it prefers moist soil with partial shade. The leaves are lemon scented.

Part Used

• Leaves

Medical Uses

Lemon balm is used as a sleep aid and for nervousness and stomachaches. In Europe, lemon balm topical cream is used to treat oral and genital herpes. Lemon balm leaves can be added to vegetable dishes, fish, and chicken.

Dosage

Tea: Pour one cup of boiling water over 1 to 2 teaspoons of finely chopped leaves and steep for 5 minutes.

Extract cream (external use): Apply standard *Melissa* 70:1 extract cream in a thick layer at the first sign of blisters four times a day up to 14 days. Also may be used on a regular basis twice a day to prevent cold sores.

Warnings

• If you are pregnant and think that you might have genital herpes, consult your health-care practitioner.
• Lemon balm does not help to prevent the spread of genital herpes in sexually active individuals.

RECIPES

LEMONADE

On a hot summer day, pick fresh lemon balm leaves. Pour 1 cup of hot water over the leaves, let sit for 10 minutes, and strain. Let the liquid cool, add ice and a little honey or turbinado sugar, and you have a refreshing cup of lemonade.

LICORICE
(Glycyrrhiza glabra)

Historical Uses

Historically, licorice has been used as a flavoring agent in candy, tobacco, and soft drinks. Licorice syrup was used as a cough remedy. For years, licorice root has been valued in Germany and China and in Ayurvedic medicine.

Growth

Licorice comes from a small shrub that grows in temperate climates.

Part Used

- Root

Major Chemical Compounds

- Glycyrrhizin
- Flavonoids
- Phenolic compounds
- Glicophenone
- Glicoisoflavone
- Phytosterols
- Coumarins (McCaleb et al., 2000)

Clinical Uses

Licorice has been used for peptic ulcer disease, canker sores, cough, and chronic fatigue syndrome (under supervision). It is used topically for eczema, psoriasis, and herpes (Graf J, 2000). It is also used for its antibacterial activity (*Chem Pharm Bull,* 2000) and its antiparasitic, antitumor, and estrogenic activity (Rafi et al., 2000). It may be used for anti-HIV effects (DeClercq, 2000).

Mechanism of Action

Licorice does not inhibit the release of gastric acid, but rather stimulates normal defense mechanisms by improving blood supply, increasing the amount and quality of substances that line the intestinal tract, and increasing the life span of cells in the intestinal tract. It possesses mineralocorticoid properties that can lead to retention of sodium and water, potassium loss, and high blood pressure (Weiss, 1988). It has phytoestrogenic effects (Horn-Ross et al., 2000). It also has antibacterial effects on methicillin-resistant and methicillin-sensitive strains of *Staphylococcus aureus* (*Chem Pharm Bull,* 2000). It has anti-HIV action from triterpene glycyrrhizin (extracted from the root of *Glycyrrhiza radix*) that may interfere with virus-cell binding (DeClercq, 2000). Glycyrrhizin has anti-inflammatory properties, blocks C5, inhibits the lytic pathway, and may prevent tissue injury (Fujisawa et al, 2000).

Dosage

Deglycyrrhizinated licorice (DGL) is the safest form of licorice because the chemical compound glycyrrhizin has been removed (McCaleb et al., 2000). Glycyrrhizin is structurally similar to cortisol, which causes adverse effects.

Tablets: Six to eight 250-mg chewable tablets daily.

Capsules: 400 to 500 mg up to 6 times daily.

Powdered root: 1 gram up to three times daily (McCaleb et al., 2000).

For peptic ulcers: Take DGL tablets, not capsules, between meals (McCaleb et al., 2000). Do not exceed dosage and do not take for more than 4 to 6 weeks (McCaleb et al., 2000).

Side Effects

Whole licorice root may raise blood glucose levels. If patient takes more than 3 grams per day for more than 6 weeks, monitoring of blood pressure and electrolytes is suggested, along with increasing potassium intake. Foods high in potassium include figs, bananas, raisins, avocado, and baked potato with skin.

Other side effects include hypertension, sodium and water retention (aldosterone-like effects), hypokalemia (Woywoldt et al., 2000; Olukoga & Donaldson, 2000; Negro et al., 2000), vision loss (Dobbins & Saul, 2000; Negro et al., 2000), and decreased libido in men (Armanini et al., 1999). Licorice acts as an adrenal stimulant in the whole plant; use DGL, the safest form of licorice (see Dosage). Licorice root in large amounts can cause Cushing's syndrome, hypokalemia, and increased toxicity of cardiac glycosides.

Contraindications

- Diabetes
- Hypertension
- Liver and kidney disease
- Hypokalemia (McGuffin et al., 1997)

Herb-Drug Interaction

Whole licorice root should not be administered with spironolactone (WHO, 1999; Miller, 1998; Blumenthal, 2000) or amiloride (Blumenthal, 2000). It may increase potassium loss when given with thiazide diuretics and laxatives, and it may interfere with or intensify the effects of digitalis glycosides (McGuffin et al., 1997).

Pregnancy and Breast-Feeding

Licorice is not recommended during pregnancy (McGuffin et al., 1997). No restrictions are known for breast-feeding (McGuffin et al., 1997).

SUMMARY OF STUDIES

Farese et al. (*1991*). Licorice-induced hypermineralocorticoidism, noted after ingesting licorice root (more than 3 g/day for more than 6 weeks) or glycyrrhizin (100 mg/day) may cause sodium and water retention, hypertension, hypokalemia, and suppression of the renin-aldosterone system through a pseudo-aldosterone action of glycyrrhetinic acid. Monitoring of blood pressure, electrolytes was suggested, along with increasing potassium intake.

REFERENCES

Armanini, D., Bonanni, G., & Palermom (1999). Reduction of serum testosterone in men by licorice. *New England Journal of Medicine, 341*(15), 1158.

Blumenthal, M. (2000). Interactions between herbs and conventional drugs: Introductory considerations. *HerbalGram, 49,* 52–63.

Craig, W. (1997). Phytochemicals: Guardians of our health. *Journal of the American Diet Association, 10* (Suppl 2), S199–204.

DeClercq, E. (2000). Current lead natural products for the chemotherapy of human immunodeficiency virus (HIV) infection. *Medicinal Research Reviews, 20*(5), 323–49.

Dobbins, K., & Saul, R. (2000) Transient visual loss after licorice ingestion. *J Neuroopthalmology, 20*(1), 38–41.

Farese, R. V., Jr., Biglieri, E. G., Shackleton, C. H., Irony, I., & Gomez-Fontes, R. (1991). Licorice-induced hypermineralocorticoidism. *New England Journal of Medicine, 325*(17), 1223–1227.

Fujisawa, Y., Sakamoto, M., Matsushita, M., Fujita, T., & Nishioka, K. (2000). Glycyrrhizin inhibits the lytic pathway of complement-possible mechanism of its anti-inflammatory effect on liver cells in viral hepatitis. *Microbiology and Immunology, 44*(9), 799–804.

Graf, J. (2000). Herbal anti-inflammatory agents for skin disease. *Skin Therapy Letter, 5*(4), 3–5.

Hatano, T., et al. (2000). Phenolic constituents of licorice. VIII. Structures of glicophenone and glico and effects of licorice phenolics on methicillin resistant *Staphylococcus aureus. Chemical and Pharmaceutical Bulletin (Tokyo), 48*(9), 1286–1292.

Horn-Ross, P., Barnes, S., Lee, M., Coward, L., Mandel, J., Koo, J., John, E, & Smith, M. (2000). Assessing phytoestrogen exposure in epidemiologic studies: development of a database. *Cancer Causes Control, 11*(4), 289–298.

McCaleb, R., Leigh, E., & Morien, K. (2000). *The Encyclopedia of Popular Herbs.* Roseville, CA: Prima Publishing.

McGuffin, M., Hobbs, C., Upton, R., & Goldberg, A. (1997) *Botanical Safety Handbook* (p. 58). New York: CRC.

Miller, L. (1998). Herbal medicinals: Selected clinical considerations focusing on known or potential drug-herb interactions. *Archives of Internal Medicine, 158,* 2200–2211. Cited in Negro, A., Rossi, E., Regolisti, G.,

& Perazzoli, F. (2000). Liquorice-induced sodium retention. Merely an acquired condition of apparent mineralocorticoid excess? A case report. *Annali Italiani di Medicina Interna: Organo Ufficiale della Società Italiana di Medicina Interna, 15*(4), 296–300.

Vickers & Zollman (1999). Herbal medicine. *British Medical Journal, 319,* 1050–1053.

Olukoga, A. & Donaldson, D. (2000) Liquorice and its health implications. *Journal of the Royal Society of Health, 120*(2), 83–89.

Rafi, M., Posen,R., Vassil, A., Ho, C., Zhang, H., Ghai, G., Lambert, G., & DiPaola, R.(2000). Modulation of bcl-2 and cytotoxicity by licochalcone-A, a novel estrogenic flavonoid. *Anticancer Research, 20*(4), 2653–2658.

Weiss, R. F. (1988). *Herbal medicine* (p. 60). Beaconsfield, England: Beaconsfield Publishers Ltd.

World Health Organization. (1999). *WHO monographs on selected medicinal plants.* Vol. 1. Geneva: The Organization.

Woywodt, A., Hermann, A., Choi, M., Goebel, U., & Luft, F. (2000). Turkish pepper (extra hot). *Postgraduate Medical Journal, 76*(897), 426–428.

NOTES

LICORICE
(Glycyrrhiza glabra)

Historical Uses

Historically, licorice has been used as a flavoring agent in candy, tobacco, and soft drinks. Licorice syrup was used as a cough remedy. For years, licorice root has been valued in Germany and China and in Ayurvedic medicine.

Growth

Licorice comes from a small shrub that grows in temperate climates.

Part Used

• Root

Medical Uses

Licorice has been used for peptic ulcer disease, canker sores, and cough. It is used topically for eczema, psoriasis, and herpes.

Dosage

Deglycyrrhizinated licorice (DGL) is the safest form of licorice because the chemical compound glycyrrhizin has been removed. Glycyrrhizin is structurally similar to cortisol, which causes adverse effects.

Tablets: Six to eight 250-mg chewable tablets daily.

Capsules: 400 to 500 mg up to 6 times daily.

Powdered root: 1 gram up to three times daily.

For peptic ulcers: Take DGL tablets, not capsules, between meals. Do not exceed dosage and do not take for more than 4 to 6 weeks.

Warnings

• Use whole licorice root only under a health-care practitioner's care.
• Whole licorice root may raise blood sugar levels, increase blood pressure, and cause other severe side effects.
• Don't take licorice root if you have diabetes, high blood pressure, liver disease, kidney disease, or low potassium.

- Don't use licorice root if you take spironolactone, amiloride, thiazide diuretics (medications that promote the flow of urine), laxatives, or heart medications.
- Licorice root isn't recommended during pregnancy or breast-feeding. Consult your health-care practitioner.

MAITAKE MUSHROOM
(Grifola frondosa)

Historical Uses

The maitake is known as the "hen of the woods" and is valued for "maintaining health and promoting longevity" (Wood, 1999).

Growth

This mushroom is cultivated in Japan and native to the northeastern part of that country.

Part Used

• Edible mushroom

Major Chemical Compound

• D-fraction, a polysaccharide

Clinical Uses

Maitake mushroom is used for anticancer effects (Chang, 1996), immune stimulation in cancer patients, and adjunct therapy for patients undergoing chemotherapy (Nanba, 1996). It is also used for patients with HIV and AIDS (Chang, 1996), high blood pressure, hyperlipidemia, weight loss, or diabetes (*Natural Medicine*, 2000).

Mechanism of Action

The D-fraction of beta-glucan has been shown to possess antitumor activity. It also lowers blood glucose and reduces weight in rats. It has immunostimulant effects (*Natural Medicine*, 2000). The most recent maitake extract is the MD-fraction, which, combined with the D-fraction, is helpful in the treatment of cancer, HIV, hyperlipidemia, hypertension, and hepatitis (Mayell, 2001).

Dosage

Standardized to D-fraction: 6 mg twice daily between meals

Liquid (1 mg/mL): for general use 5 to 6 drops three times daily between meals (*Natural Medicine*, 2000).

199

Side Effects

Maitake mushroom lowers blood glucose levels. If stomach upset occurs, patient may take with food.

Contraindications

- Use cautiously in diabetic patients because of herb's hypoglycemic effect (*Natural Medicine*, 2000).

Herb-Drug Interactions

None are known.

Pregnancy and Breast-Feeding

No restrictions are known (McGuffin et al., 1997).

SUMMARY OF STUDIES

Most studies involving animals show weight loss and lowering of blood pressure, blood glucose levels, and lipid levels. No recent clinical studies in humans are available.

Chang (*1996*). In this review, edible mushrooms such as maitake mushrooms were found to contain functional "nutraceutical" or medicinal properties that benefit the immune system, lower lipids, and have antitumor properties without toxic effecs.

Kubo & Nanba (*1996*). In a randomized clinical trial with rats that were fed maitake mushroom dried powder and others that were fed cholesterol, the results concluded that maitake mushrooms alter lipid metabolism.

Kabir & Kimura (*1989*). After 8 weeks, hypertensive rats fed maitake mushrooms showed a reduction in high blood pressure when compared with control rats.

REFERENCES

Chang, R. (1996). Functional properties of edible mushrooms. *Nutrition Review, 54*(11, Pt. 2), S91–S93.

Kabir, Y., & Kimura, S. (1989). Dietary mushrooms reduce blood pressure in spontaneously hypertensive rats (SHR). *Journal of Nutritional Science and Vitaminology* (*Tokyo*), *35*(1), 91–94.

Kubo, K., & Nanba, H. (1996). The effect of maitake mushrooms on liver and serum lipids. *Alternative Therapies in Health and Medicine, 2*(5), 62–66.

Mayell, M. (2001). Maitake extracts and their therapeutic potential. *Alternative Medicine Review, 6*(1), 48–60.

McGuffin, M., Hobbs, C., Upton, R., & Goldberg, A. (1997) *Botanical safety handbook.* New York: CRC.

Nanba, H. (February/March 1996). Maitake D-fraction healing and preventing potentials for cancer. *Townsend Letter for Doctors and Patients,* 84–85.

Natural Medicines Comprehensive Database. (2000). *Pharmacist's Letter and Prescriber's Letter* (pp. 699–700). Therapeutic Research Faculty.

Wood, R. (1999). *The new whole foods encyclopedia.* New York: Penguin, p. 159.

NOTES

NOTES

MAITAKE MUSHROOM
(Grifola frondosa)

Historical Uses

The maitake is known as the "hen of the woods" and is valued for "maintaining health and promoting longevity."

Growth

This mushroom is cultivated in Japan and is native to the northeastern part of that country.

Part Used

• Edible mushroom

Medical Uses

Maitake mushroom is used for anticancer effects, stimulation of the immune system in cancer patients, and as supportive therapy for patients undergoing chemotherapy or patients with HIV or AIDS, high blood pressure, hyperlipidemia, weight loss, or diabetes.

Dosage

Standardized to D-fraction: 6 mg twice daily between meals.

Liquid (1 mg/mL): for general use 5 to 6 drops three times daily between meals.

Warnings

• Lowers blood sugar levels.
• If stomach upset occurs, take with food.
• Don't use maitake mushroom if you have diabetes.

MARIGOLD (CALENDULA)

(Calendula officinalis)

Historical Uses

Calendula infusion has been used for breaking fevers and treating conjunctivitis. It has also been used for its antispasmodic and stimulant effects. The tincture has been applied to sprains. It was used during the Civil War as an antiseptic for wounds. It is also called pot marigold.

Growth

A member of the Asteraceae family, calendula can be grown in herb gardens. It is an annual plant with yellowish-orange petals that open and close with the sun. Plant it in late spring in temperate climates; it prefers well-drained soil. Pick the flower heads when they open and dry them on paper in a warm, dark place. Separate the petals from the head and store them in dark jars (Weiss, 1985). They can be used to make calendula cream or oil.

Part Used

- Flower petals

Major Chemical Compounds

- Carotenoids
- Volatile oil
- Mucilage
- Saponins (Tyler, 1993)

Clinical Uses

Calendula is used externally for skin irritations and wound healing (Patrick et al., 1996; Garg & Sharma, 1992) and for juvenile acne (Verbuta & Cojocaru, 1996). It is approved for use by the German Commission E for wound healing (Blumenthal et al., 2000).

Mechanism of Action

Calendula has anti-inflammatory and wound-healing properties; the mechanism is unknown (Tyler, 1993). It has been shown to possess anti-HIV properties (Kalvatchev et al., 1997).

Dosage

Apply calendula ointment or cream topically to wounds and dry, irritated skin. Calendula soap is also available and may be used to help treat acne.

Side Effects

None are known.

Contraindications

• None are known.

Herb-Drug Interactions

None are known.

Pregnancy and Breast-Feeding

No restrictions are known for pregnant and breast-feeding women (Blumenthal, et al., 2000; McGuffin, et al., 1997).

SUMMARY OF STUDIES

Several studies using calendula externally are available in the homeopathic literature.

REFERENCES

Blumenthal, M., Goldberg, A., & Brinckmann, J. (Eds.). (2000). *Herbal medicine expanded Commission E monographs.* Austin, TX: American Botanical Council; Newton, MA: Integrative Medicine Communications.

Fox, H. (1953.) *The Years in My Herb Garden* (p. 116). New York: Macmillan Company.

Garg, S., & Sharma, S. N. (1992). Development of medicated aerosol dressings of chlorhexidine acetate with hemostatics. *Pharmazie, 47*(12), 924–926.

Kalvatchev, Z., Walder, R., & Garzaro, D. (1997). Anti-HIV activity of extracts from *Calendula officinalis* flowers. *Biomedicine and Pharmacotherapy, 51*(4), 176–180.

McGuffin, M., Hobbs, C., Upton, R., & Goldberg, A. (1997) *Botanical Safety Handbook.* New York: CRC.

Patrick, K., Kumar, S., Edwardson, P., & Hutchinson, J. J. (1996). Induction of vascularisation by an aqueous extract of the flowers of *Calendula officinalis. Phytomedicine, 3,* 11–18.

Patrick K, Kumar S, Edwardson P, Hutchinson JJ (1996). Induction of vascularization by an aqueous extract of the flowers of *Calendula officinalis. Phytomed* 3:11–18.

Tyler, V. (1993). *The honest herbal.* Binghamton, NY: Pharmaceutical Products Press.

Verbuta, A., & Cojocaru, I. (1996). Research to achieve a homeopathic lotion. *Revista Medico-Chirurgicala a Societatii de Medici si Naturalisti din Iasi, 100*(1–2), 172–174.

Weiss, G., & Weiss, S. (1985). *Growing and using the healing herbs* (pp. 97–98). Emmaus, PA: Rodale Press.

NOTES

MARIGOLD (CALENDULA)
(Calendula officinalis)

Historical Uses

Calendula infusion has been used for breaking fevers and treating conjunctivitis. It has also been used for its antispasmodic and stimulant effects. The tincture has been applied to sprains. It was used during the Civil War as an antiseptic for wounds. It is also called pot marigold.

Growth

A member of the Asteraceae family, calendula can be grown in herb gardens. It is an annual plant with yellowish-orange petals that open and close with the sun. Plant it in late spring in temperate climates; it prefers well-drained soil. Pick the flower heads when they open and dry them on paper in a warm, dark place. Separate the petals from the head and store them in dark jars. They can be used to make calendula cream or oil.

Part Used

• Flower petals

Medical Uses

Calendula is used externally for skin irritations and wound healing.

Dosage

Apply calendula ointment or cream two to three times a day to wounds and dry, irritated skin. Calendula soap is also available and may be used to help treat acne.

Warnings

• None are known.

RECIPES

Calendula petals have a nutty flavor and may be used to color butter and puddings.

CALENDULA OIL AND SALVE

Place 2 cups of oil (olive, safflower, canola, vitamin E, or almond oil) in a glass or enameled double boiler. Place 3 ounces of calendula flowers in the oil and simmer for up to 30 minutes. Don't boil; if you see smoke or bubbling of the entire mixture, the oil is too hot. After simmering, strain through cheesecloth and pour the oil into small jars. Use the oil on dry skin. To make a salve for dry skin, reheat 1 cup of calendula oil and add ¼ cup of beeswax. Cool the salve and place it in jars with lids. Label and date the mixture; refrigerate it to maximize shelf life.

MILK THISTLE
(Silybum marianum)

Historical Uses

Milk thistle has been used traditionally for liver complaints.

Growth

A member of the aster family, milk thistle is native to southern and western Europe and some parts of the U.S.

Part Used

• Fruits, known as achenes (Tyler, 1993)

Major Chemical Compounds

• Silymarin
• Silibinin

Clinical Uses

Milk thistle improves liver function tests and reverses mushroom (*Amanita phalloides*) poisoning if given within 24 hours after ingestion of the mushroom. It can also be used for chemical-induced liver damage, cirrhosis, and viral hepatitis. Silibinin may be useful in prostate cancer (Zi & Agarwal, 1999). It is approved by the German Commission E for dyspepsia, liver damage, and liver disease (Blumenthal et al., 2000).

Mechanism of Action

This herb has antioxidant, hepatoprotective, and hepatorestorative properties (Palasciano, G., et al., 1995; Fintelmann, V., 1986). It also increases the gluthione content of liver, inhibits leukotrienes, and stimulates protein synthesis. Silibinin, an antioxidant in milk thistle, has been shown to inhibit prostate cancer cells, although the mechanism of action is still unknown (Zi et al., 2000).

Dosage

Standardized capsules or tablets: 420 mg divided into two to three doses a day (McCaleb et al., 2000). Results are usually seen after 6 to 8 weeks and should be verified by liver function tests (Ottariano, 1999). After 6 to 8 weeks, dosage may be reduced to 280 mg daily (McCaleb et al., 2000).

Tea: Silymarin is poorly soluble in water and therefore should not be taken in tea form (Tyler, 1993).

Side Effects

The patient may develop loose stools at high doses.

Contraindications

• Monitor blood glucose levels in diabetic patients. Standard anti-hyperglycemic medications may need to be reduced. (McCaleb et al., 2000).

Herb-Drug Interactions

Monitor blood glucose levels in patients taking diabetic medications (McCaleb et al., 2000).

Pregnancy and Breast-Feeding

There are no restrictions (McGuffin et al., 1997). However, use cautiously in pregnant patients because the herb has a laxative effect (Ottariano, 1999).

SUMMARY OF STUDIES

Palasciano et al. (*1995*). Fifteen subjects receiving butyrophenones and phenothiazines were also given 400 mg b.i.d. of concentrated extracts from the fruits of milk thistle. Results: milk thistle protected the liver from the adverse effects of these drugs.

Fintelmann (1986). Results: Milk thistle reduced the hepatotoxic effects of phenytoin.

REFERENCES

Blumenthal, M., Goldberg, A., & Brinckmann, J. (Eds.). (2000). *Herbal medicine expanded Commission E monographs* (pp. 257–261). Austin, TX: American Botanical Council; Newton, MA: Integrative Medicine Communications.

Fintelmann, V. (1986). Toxic metabolic liver damage and its treatment. *Z Phytother, 3,* 65–73.

McCaleb, R., Leigh, E., & Morien, K. (2000). *The encyclopedia of popular herbs.* Roseville, CA: Prima Publishing.

McGuffin, M., Hobbs, C., Upton, R., & Goldberg, A. (1997). *Botanical safety handbook* (p. 107). New York: CRC.

Ottariano, S. (1999). *Medicinal herbal therapy: A pharmacist's viewpoint.* North Hampton, NH: Nicolin Fields Publishing.

Palasciano, G., et al. (1994). The effect of silymarin on plasma levels of malon-dialdehyde in patients receiving long-term treatment with psychotropic drugs. *Current Therapeutic Research, 55,* 537–545.

Tyler, V. (1993). *The honest herbal.* Binghamton, NY: Pharmaceutical Products Press.

Zi, X., & Agarwal, R. (1999). Silibinin decreases prostate-specific antigen with cell growth inhibition via GI arrest, leading to differentiation of prostate carcinoma cells: Implications for prostate cancer intervention. *Proceedings of the National Academy of Sciences of the United States of America, 96*(13), 7490–7495.

Zi, X., Zhang, J., Agarwal, R., & Pollack, M. (2000). Silibinin up-regulates insulin-like growth factor-binding protein 3 expression and inhibits proliferation of androgen-independent prostate cancer cells. *Cancer Research, 60*(20), 5617–5620.

NOTES

NOTES

MILK THISTLE
(Silybum marianum)

Historical Uses

Milk thistle has been used traditionally for liver complaints.

Growth

A member of the aster family, milk thistle is native to southern and western Europe and some parts of United States.

Part Used

• Fruits, known as achenes

Medical Uses

Milk thistle improves liver function tests and helps to counteract mushroom (*Amanita phalloides*) poisoning if taken within 24 hours after ingestion of the mushroom. It can also be used for chemical-induced liver damage, cirrhosis, and viral hepatitis.

Dosage

Standardized capsules or tablets: 420 mg divided into two to three doses a day. Results are usually seen after 6 to 8 weeks and should be verified by liver function tests. After 6 to 8 weeks, dosage may be reduced to 280 mg daily.

Warnings

• Milk thistle is poorly soluble in water and therefore should not be taken in tea form.
• Milk thistle may cause loose stools at high doses.
• Monitor your blood sugar levels closely if you have diabetes or take an antidiabetic medication.
• Avoid use of this herb if you are pregnant or breast-feeding.

NETTLE
(Urtica dioica)

Historical Uses

Nettle is the Anglo-Saxon word for "needle." In folklore, nettle was used as a footbath for rheumatism, a spring tonic, a diuretic, and a remedy for asthma.

Growth

Nettle grows 2 to 3 feet high and has dark green leaves with stinging hairs. Touching or brushing against the leaves sometimes causes a severe local irritation.

Parts Used

- Leaves
- Roots

Major Chemical Compounds

- Flavonoids
- Acetylcholine
- Histamine
- Serotonin
- Chlorophyll
- Carotenoids
- High amounts of iron, calcium, vitamin C, and silica.

Clinical Uses

Nettle is used for allergy symptoms and anemia. It also is used to prevent hair loss, stimulate hair growth, promote weight loss, and strengthen the liver. It is used as a nutritive tea for pregnant and breast-feeding women. It can also be used for arthritis pain (Chrubasik et al., 1997) and for its anti-HIV effects (DeClercq, 2000).

Mechanism of Action

This herb has antihistamine and diuretic effects. It increases production of breast milk. It has antiprostatic, androgenic, keratogenetic, and testosteronigenic effects (Duke, 2000). Its anti-HIV effects result from a virus-cell fusion process of N-acteyl-glucosamine-specific lectin (DeClercq, 2000).

Dosage

Do not administer raw nettle.

Tincture: 2 to 5 mL (1/2 to 1 teaspoon) three times a day (Yarnell, E., 1998).

Decoction for root: 1 teaspoon dried root in 1 cup water, boiled for 10 to 15 minutes and then strained and drunk.

Infusion for nettle leaves: 2 to 5 grams (2 to 3 teaspoons) of leaves in 150 mL of boiling water, steeped for about 5 to 10 minutes. Tea may be administered three times a day.

Side Effects

Nettle may increase blood glucose levels slightly (Roman Ramos et al., 1992).

Contraindications

• Nettle is contraindicated in patients who are allergic to it.

Herb-Drug Interactions

Monitor blood glucose levels in patients who take diabetic medications (Roman Ramos et al., 1992). Taking herb with diclofenac may increase anti-inflammatory effects (Chrubasik, S., et al., 1997).

Pregnancy and Breast-Feeding

No restrictions are known (McGuffin et al., 1997).

 # SUMMARY OF STUDIES

Marks et al. (2000). This American study was a controlled, 6-month trial using 44 subjects who took a blend of saw palmetto extract, nettle root extract, and pumpkin seed oil (Nutrilite product of Amway) for symptoms of benign prostatic hyperplasia. Results: Symptoms were improved, but not to a statistically significant level. The growth of prostate tissue was slowed via a nonhormonal mechanism without affecting serum prostate-specific antigen levels.

Chrubasik et al. (1997). This open, randomized study included 40 patients with acute arthritis. Of the 40, 20 patients took diclofenac (Voltaren) 200 mg and 20 patients took 50 mg of diclofenac with 50 grams of stewed nettle leaf. Results: A combination of 50 grams of nettle leaf with 20 mg diclofenac was just as effective in relieving pain as the full dose of diclofenac.

REFERENCES

Chrubasik, S., Enderlein, W., Bauer, R., & Grabner, W. (1997). Evidence for antirheumatic effectiveness of *Herba urticae dioicae* in acute arthritis: A pilot study. *Phytomedicine, 4*(2), 105–108.

DeClercq, E. (2000). Current lead natural products for the chemotherapy of human immunodeficiency virus (HIV) infection. *Medicinal Research Reviews, 20*(5), 323–349.

Duke, J. (2000) Phytochemical and Ethnobotanical Database at the Agricultural Research Services.

Marks, L. S., Partin, A. W., Epstein, J. I., Tyler, V. E., Simon, I., Macairan, M. L., Chan, T. L., Dorey, F. J., Garris, J. B., Veltri, R. W., Santos, P. B., Stonebrook, K. A., & de Kernion, J. B. (2000). Effects of a saw palmetto herbal blend in men with symptomatic benign prostatic hyperplasia. *Journal of Urology, 163*(5), 1451–1456.

McGuffin, M., Hobbs, C., Upton, R., & Goldberg, A. (1997) *Botanical Safety Handbook* (p. 119). New York: CRC.

Roman Ramos, R., Alarcon-Aguilar, F., Lara-Lemus, A., & Flores-Saenz, J. (1992). Hypoglycemic effect of plants used in Mexico as antidiabetics. *Archives of Medical Research, 23*(1):59–64.

Yarnell, E. (June 1998). Stinging nettle: a modern view of an ancient healing plant. *Alternative and Complementary Therapies,* 180–186.

NOTES

NETTLE
⟨Urtica dioica⟩

Historical Uses

Nettle is the Anglo-Saxon word for "needle." In folklore, nettle was used as a footbath for rheumatism, a spring tonic, a diuretic, and a remedy for asthma.

Growth

Nettle grows 2 to 3 feet high and has dark green leaves with stinging hairs. Touching or brushing against the leaves sometimes causes a severe local irritation.

Parts Used

- Leaves
- Roots

Medical Uses

Nettle is used for allergy symptoms and anemia. It also is used to prevent hair loss, stimulate hair growth, promote weight loss, and strengthen the liver. It is used as a nutritive tea for pregnant and breast-feeding women. It can also be used for arthritis pain.

Dosage

Do not take raw nettle.

Tincture: 2 to 5 mL ($^1/_2$ to 1 teaspoon) three times a day.

Decoction for root: 1 teaspoon of dried root in 1 cup of water, boiled for 10 to 15 minutes and then strained and drunk.

Infusion for nettle leaves: 2 to 5 grams (2 to 3 teaspoons) of leaves in 150 mL of boiling water, steeped for about 5 to 10 minutes. Tea may be administered three times a day.

Warnings

- Nettle may slightly increase blood glucose levels. Monitor your blood glucose levels closely if you have diabetes or take an antidiabetic medication.
- Don't use nettle if you are allergic to it.
- Don't use nettle if you take diclofenac.

RECIPES

Prepare nettle as you would spinach. You also may sauté young nettle shoots with onions and carrots or add nettle to soups. **Do not eat raw nettle.**

HAIR RINSE

To prevent hair loss if you have cancer, finely chop ½ lb fresh nettle leaves. Boil in 1 pint water and 1 pint vinegar for 20 minutes. Strain and place in bottles to use as a hair rinse.

SPRING TONIC

Combine equal parts of cooked nettle leaves and dandelion leaves for a wonderful spring tonic to purify the blood. Drink 3 cups a day to help combat anemia.

OATS

(Avena sativa)

Historical Uses

Oats have been used to stabilize blood glucose levels, soothe the nervous and digestive systems, reduce cravings for cigarettes, and reduce cholesterol levels. Used externally, they help stop itching from conditions as chickenpox and shingles.

Growth

Oats are grown as a crop in sunny, well-drained, fertile soil. Threshing separates the grains, which are then dehusked and rolled for cereals (Bown, 1995). Seeds are milled from the cultivated plant.

Part Used

• Seeds

Major Chemical Compounds

• Alkaloid
• Glycosides
• Fixed oils
• Iron
• Zinc

Clinical Uses

Besides their nutritive value, oats are an adaptogenic grain (they help with stress). They also lower cholesterol (Onning et al., 1999) and help to relieve menopausal symptoms. Oats are used externally for eczema, psoriasis, chickenpox, and shingles (herpes zoster). Oats and a low-calorie diet help to lower blood pressure and improve lipid profiles (Saltzman et al., 2001). Oatstraw (dried, threshed leaf and stem of the oat plant) is approved by the German Commission E for "topical applications in herbal baths for inflammation and seborrheic skin diseases with pruritus" (Blumenthal et al., 2000).

Mechanism of Action

Oats have a high vitamin and mineral content that helps to relax the central nervous system.

Dosage

Use externally in oatmeal baths and soaps. Safe to consume in foods.

Oatmeal bath: 100 grams of oatstraw added to warm bath water (Blumenthal et al., 2000).

Side Effects

None are known.

Contraindications

• None are known.

Herb-Drug Interactions

None are known.

Pregnancy and Breast-Feeding

No restrictions are known.

SUMMARY OF STUDIES

Onning et al. (1999). This randomized, controlled, double-blind study included 66 men who consumed 0.75 L/day of oat milk or rice milk. Results: Oat milk significantly lowered serum total cholesterol and decreased low-density lipoprotein levels, an effect that was more pronounced if the starting cholesterol value was higher. Serum triglycerides remained the same, as did high-density lipoprotein levels.

Saltzman et al. (2001). This randomized controlled study of 43 adults was an 8-week study to determine a diet that decreased cardiovascular risk. A low-calorie diet that included oats showed greater improvement in lowering blood pressure and improved lipid profiles.

REFERENCES

Bown, D. (1995). *The Herb Society of America encyclopedia of herbs and their uses.* New York: Dorling Kindersley Publishing.

Blumenthal, M., Goldberg, A., & Brinckmann, J. (Eds.). (2000). *Herbal medicine expanded Commission E monographs* (pp. 281–282). Austin, TX: American Botanical Council; Newton, MA: Integrative Medicine Communications.

Onning, G., Wallmark, A., Persson, M., Akesson, B., Elm Stahl, S., & Oste, R. (1999). Consumption of oat milk for 5 weeks lowers serum cholesterol and LDL cholesterol in free-living men with moderate hypercholesterolemia. *Annals of Nutrition and Metabolism, 43*(5), 301–309.

Saltzman, E., Das, K., Lichtenstein, A. H., Dallal, G. E., Corrales, A., Schaefer, E. J., Greenberg, A. S., & Roberts, S. B. (2001). An oat-containing hypocaloric diet reduces systolic blood pressure and improves lipid profile beyond effects of weight loss in men and women. *Journal of Nutrition, 131*(5), 1465–1470.

Wood, R. (1999). *The new whole foods encyclopedia* (pp. 233–234). New York: Penguin Press.

NOTES

NOTES

OATS
(Avena sativa)

Historical Uses

Oats have been used to stabilize blood glucose levels, soothe the nervous and digestive systems, reduce cravings for cigarettes, and reduce cholesterol levels. Used externally, they help stop itching from conditions such as chickenpox and shingles.

Growth

Oats are grown as a crop in sunny, well-drained, fertile soil. Threshing separates the grains, which are then dehusked and rolled for cereals. Seeds are milled from the cultivated plant.

Part Used

• Seeds

Medical Uses

Besides their nutritive value, oats are an adaptogenic grain (they help with stress). They also lower cholesterol and help to relieve menopausal symptoms. Oats are used externally for eczema, psoriasis, chickenpox, and shingles (herpes zoster). Oatstraw (dried, threshed leaf and stem of the oat plant) may be used in herbal baths for inflammation and seborrheic skin conditions with itching.

Dosage

Use externally in oatmeal baths and soaps. Oats are safe to consume in foods.

Oatmeal bath: 100 grams of oatstraw added to warm bath water (Blumenthal et al., 2000).

Warnings

• None are known.

RECIPES

Oatmeal contains unsaturated fat, protein, sodium, and vitamin E. It is used in hot and cold cereals, "natural" snack bars, and casseroles as a substitute for rice.

HERBAL BATH FOR DRY SKIN

Mix 1 quart of nonfat milk powder with ½ cup of finely ground oatmeal. Add ¼ cup of crushed chamomile flowers. Mix with warm bath water or put into herbal bath sack and float the sack in the bath. Soak for about 15 minutes. Rinse and dry.

HERBAL BATH FOR RELAXATION

Place 3 tablespoons of lavender flowers and 3 tablespoons of ground oatmeal into a cotton bath sack and let the sack float in the water as you bathe. Or hang the sack on the faucet while you fill the tub. Light candles and play soft, soothing music while you soak.

PEPPERMINT
(Mentha x piperita)

Historical Uses

Peppermint has been used historically for indigestion, colic, and fevers.

Growth

This perennial aromatic herb of the mint family can be grown as a houseplant or in an herb garden. It spreads easily in a garden.

Part Used

• Leaves

Major Chemical Compounds

• Volatile oil made up of menthol, menthone, and menthyl acetate

Clinical Uses

Peppermint is given for colds, fevers, and gastrointestinal complaints. Peppermint oil capsules have improved symptoms of irritable bowel syndrome (Kline et al., 2001).

Mechanism of Action

This herb has carmative (gas-relieving) and antispasmodic effects because it blocks calcium and decreases hypercontractility of intestinal smooth muscle (Miclefield et al., 2000). Menthol has a choleretic effect.

Dosage

Tea (infusion): 1 to 2 teaspoons of dried leaves in 8 ounces of boiling water, steeped for 5 minutes. Cover the cup to prevent volatile oils from escaping. Drink three times daily.

Side Effects

Peppermint may cause hypersensitivity reactions and contact dermatitis.

Contraindications

• Peppermint is contraindicated in patients with gallstones.

- Peppermint may reduce or negate the beneficial effects of homeopathic remedies. Consult a homeopathic practitioner before taking peppermint along with these remedies.

Herb-Drug Interactions

None are known.

Pregnancy and breast-feeding

No restrictions are known (McGuffin et al., 1997).

 # SUMMARY OF STUDIES

Most studies are done with peppermint oil capsules, not peppermint leaf.

Kline et al. (2001). This randomized, double-blind, controlled, multicenter study of 42 children with a diagnosis of irritable bowel syndrome showed improvement in 75 percent of those who received peppermint oil capsules for 2 weeks.

May et al. (2000). This randomized, controlled trial using one capsule twice daily of 90 mg peppermint oil and 50 mg caraway oil (Enteroplant) in 96 patients with a diagnosis of functional dyspepsia over 28 days resulted in a positive risk-beneft ratio and was well tolerated.

REFERENCES

Blumenthal, M., Busse, W., Goldberg, A., Gruenwald, J., Hall, T., Riggins, C., & Rister, R. (Eds.). (1998). *The complete German Commission E monographs: Therapeutic guide to herbal medicines.* (S. Klein & R. Rister, Trans.). Austin, TX: American Botanical Council; Newton, MA: Integrative Medicine Communications.

Kline, R. M., Kline, J. J., Di Palma, J., & Barbero, G. J. (2001). Enteric-coated, pH-dependent peppermint oil capsules for the treatment of irritable bowel syndrome in children. *Journal of Pediatrics, 138*(1), 125–128.

May, B., Kohler, S., & Schneider, B. (2000). Efficacy and tolerability of a fixed combination of peppermint oil and caraway oil in patients suffering from functional dyspepsia. *Alimentary Pharmacology and Therapeutics, 14*(12), 1671–1677.

McGuffin, M., Hobbs, C., Upton, R., & Goldberg, A. (1997) *Botanical Safety Handbook.* New York: CRC.

Micklefield, G., Grieving, I., & May, B. (2000). Effects of peppermint oil and caraway oil on gastroduodenal motility. *Phytotherapy Research, 14*(1), 20–23.

Wood, R. (1999). *The new whole foods encyclopedia.* New York: Penguin Press.

NOTES

PEPPERMINT
(Mentha x piperita)

Historical Uses

Peppermint has been used historically for indigestion, colic, and fevers.

Growth

This perennial aromatic herb of the mint family can be grown as a houseplant or in an herb garden. It spreads easily in a garden.

Part Used

• Leaves

Medical Uses

Peppermint is used for colds, fevers, and gastrointestinal complaints.

Dosage

Tea (infusion): 1 to 2 teaspoons of dried leaves in 8 ounces of boiling water, steeped for 5 minutes. Cover the cup to prevent volatile oils from escaping. Drink three times daily.

Warnings

• Peppermint may cause allergic reactions and rash.
• Don't take peppermint if you have gallstones.
• Peppermint may interfere with homeopathic remedies. If you take such a remedy, consult your homeopathic practitioner.

RED RASPBERRY
(Rubus idaeus)

Historical Uses

Raspberry leaves have been used as a folk remedy for mouth sores, irritated mucous membranes, and diarrhea. Herbalists have sometimes called the red raspberry the herb for pregnancy.

Growth

The raspberry plant is a thorny bush that grows to about 6 feet high. It originated in Europe and Asia and grows in temperate areas. It resembles but should not be confused with the blackberry plant.

Parts Used

- Leaves
- Fruit

Major Chemical Compounds

- Vitamins A, B, C, and E
- Calcium
- Phosphorus
- Iron
- Fragarine
- Ellagic acid

Clinical Uses

Modern use is based on the traditional uses of raspberry for mouth sores, irritated mucous membranes, and diarrhea. It may also inhibit the growth of cancer cells (Khalsa, 2000). In a survey of Certified Nursing Midwives who used herbal preparations, 63 percent stated that they used red raspberry leaf to stimulate labor (McFarlin et al., 1999).

Mechanism of Action

Ellagic acid has antimutagenic, anticarcinogenic, antibacterial, and antiviral properties (Khalsa, 2000). The astringent properties, which are helpful in alleviating mouth sores and diarrhea, result from the tannin content (Tyler, 1993). Tannins cause vaso-

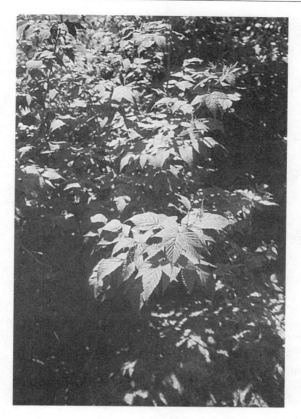

constriction and have anti-inflammatory properties when applied externally (*Natural Medicines,* 2000).

Dosage

Tea (*infusion*): 2 teaspoons of raspberry leaves in 1 cup of boiling water, steeped for 5 minutes. Strain and drink up to three times a day (*Natural Medicines,* 2000).

Gargle: Tea infusion may be used as a gargle for irritated mucous membranes.

Lip balm: Made with red raspberry leaves and lemon balm and used for cold sores on lips.

Side Effects

Raspberry may cause allergic reactions.

Contraindications

• None are known.

Herb-Drug Interactions

None are known.

Pregnancy and Breast-Feeding

No restrictions are known (McGuffin et al., 1997).

 # SUMMARY OF STUDIES

Current studies in progress at the Hollings Cancer Center of the Medical University of South Carolina are looking at the consumption of 1 cup (150 grams) of red raspberries a day and its potential to slow the growth of abnormal colon cells and prevent development of human papilloma virus. Another study by Nixon is looking at red raspberries in prevention of cervical cancer (Khalsa, 2000).

REFERENCES

Khalsa, K. (September/October 2000). Red raspberries may prevent cancer. *Herbs for Health,* 16.

McFarlin, B., Gibson, M., O'Rear, J., & Harmon, P. (May–June, 1999). A national survey of herbal preparation use by nurse-midwives for labor stimulation: Review of the literature and recommendations for practice. *Journal of Nurse Midwifery, 44*(3), 183–188, 205–216.

McGuffin, M., Hobbs, C., Upton, R., & Goldberg, A. (1997) *Botanical Safety Handbook.* New York: CRC.

Natural Medicines Comprehensive Database. (2000). *Pharmacist's Letter and Prescriber's Letter* (pp. 885–886). Therapeutic Research Faculty.

Tyler, V. (1993). *The honest herbal* (pp. 257–258). Binghamton, NY: Pharmaceutical Products Press.

NOTES

RED RASPBERRY
(Rubus idaeus)

Historical Uses

Raspberry leaves have been used as a folk remedy for mouth sores, irritated mucous membranes, and diarrhea. Herbalists have sometimes called the red raspberry the herb for pregnancy.

Growth

The raspberry plant is a thorny bush that grows to about 6 feet high. It originated in Europe and Asia and grows in temperate areas. It resembles but should not be confused with the blackberry plant.

Part Used

- Leaves
- Fruit

Medical Uses

Modern use is based on the traditional uses of raspberry for mouth sores, irritated mucous membranes, and diarrhea. It may also inhibit the growth of cancer cells.

Dosage

Tea (infusion): Place 2 teaspoons of raspberry leaves in one cup of boiling water and steep for 5 minutes. Strain and drink up to three times a day.

Gargle: Tea infusion may be used as a gargle for irritated mucous membranes.

Lip balm: Made with red raspberry leaves and lemon balm and used for cold sores on lips (see recipe).

Warnings

- Raspberry may cause allergic reactions.

RECIPES

RED RASPBERRY LIP BALM

Place 2 cups oil (olive, safflower, or canola) in a glass or enameled double boiler. Place 3 ounces of red raspberry leaf (combined with lemon balm if desired) in the oil and simmer for up to 30 minutes. Do not boil; if you see smoke or bubbling of the entire mixture, the oil is too hot. Then place ⅓ cup of beeswax into the top of a double boiler. As it begins to melt, add the herbal oil and stir. Allow the mixture to cool, and pour it into small containers. Label and date the containers and store them in the refrigerator to maximize shelf life.

REISHI MUSHROOM

(Ganoderma lucidum)

Historical Uses

Historically in China and Japan, the reishi mushroom has been called "the mushroom of immortality" because of its medicinal properties, which stimulate the immune system.

Growth

This fungus is a member of the Ganoderma family of fungi.

Parts used

- Fruiting body
- Mycelium

Major Chemical Compounds

- Polysaccharides

Clinical Uses

Reishi mushroom is used to support the immune system, usually for prevention and long-term use (Wasser & Weis, 1999; Yoshida et al., 1997). It may lower blood glucose levels (Marles & Farnsworth, 1995).

Mechanism of Action

Polysaccharides bind to specialized receptor sites on macrophages and natural killer cells, which send out chemical signals to fight off infection (Roundtree, 2000).

Dosage

Crude dried mushroom: 1.5 to 9 grams daily by mouth.

Reishi powder: 1 to 1.5 grams daily by mouth.

Reishi tincture: 1 mL daily by mouth (*Natural Medicines*, 2000).

Side Effects

Prolonged use of reishi mushroom (more than 3 months) has resulted in infrequent reports of dry mouth and stomach upset (McGuffin et al., 1997). It may prolong bleeding times.

Contraindications

• None are known.

Herb-Drug Interactions

Reishi mushroom is contraindicated for patients who take anticoagulants or anti-hypertensive medications.

Pregnancy and Breast-Feeding

No restrictions are known (McGuffin et al., 1997).

SUMMARY OF STUDIES

Limited clinical studies are available.

REFERENCES

International Journal of Cancer. May help the body fight tumors by stimulating immune cells. *70*(6), 669–705.

Marles, R., & Farnsworth, N. (1995). Antidiabetic plants and their active constituents. *Phytomedicine, 2*(2), 137–189.

McGuffin, M., Hobbs, C., Upton, R., & Goldberg, A. (1997) *Botanical Safety Handbook.* New York: CRC.

Natural Medicines Comprehensive Database. (2000). *Pharmacist's Letter and Prescriber's Letter* (pp. 894–895). Therapeutic Research Faculty.

Roundtree, R. (November/December 2000). Immune suppressants and herbal medicines. *Herbs for Health,* 26–27.

Wasser, S., & Weis, A. (1999). Therapeutic effects of substances occurring in higher *Basidiomycetes* mushrooms: a modern perspective. *Critical Review of Immunology, 19*(1), 65–96.

Yoshida, Y., Wang, M., Liu, J., Shan, B., & Yamashita, U. (1997). Immunomodulating activity of Chinese medicinal herbs and *Oldenlandra diffusa* in particular. *International Immunopharmacology, 19*(7), 359–370.

NOTES

REISHI MUSHROOM
(Ganoderma lucidum)

Historical Uses

Historically in China and Japan, the reishi mushroom has been called "the mushroom of immortality" because of its medicinal properties, which stimulate the immune system.

Growth

This fungus is a member of the Ganoderma family of fungi.

Part Used

- Fruiting body
- Mycelium

Medical Uses

Reishi mushroom is used to support the immune system, usually for prevention and long-term use. It may lower blood sugar levels.

Dosage

Crude dried mushroom: 1.5 to 9 grams daily by mouth.

Reishi powder: 1 to 1.5 grams daily by mouth.

Reishi tincture: 1 mL daily by mouth.

Warnings

- Prolonged use of reishi mushroom (more than 3 months) has resulted in infrequent reports of dry mouth and stomach upset.
- Reishi mushroom may increase the risk of bleeding. Don't use it if you take a blood thinner or a medication for high blood pressure.

ST. JOHN'S WORT

(Hypericum perforatum)

Historical Uses

St. John's wort was used by the ancient Greeks for sciatica and nervous disorders. It has also been used as a popular folk remedy for neuralgias, sciatica, burns or bruises involving nerve damage, sprains, emotional disorders, wounds, and tennis elbow.

Growth

This plant grows in fields and on roadsides throughout the United States. It reaches about 1 to 3 feet in height, and its yellow flowers bloom from June to September.

Parts Used

- Aerial (above-ground) parts

Major Chemical Compounds

- Hypericin
- Hyperforin
- Flavonoids

Clinical Uses

St. John's wort is given orally for mild to moderate depression, not for severe depression or bipolar disorder. It can be used externally for tennis elbow, sprains, and strains. It is approved by the German Commission E to be used "internally for depressive moods, anxiety, externally for acute and contused injuries, myalgia, and first-degree burns" (Blumenthal et al., 2000).

St. John's wort is at least as safe as, and possibly safer than, fluoxetine (Prozac) (Schrader, (2000); moclobemide, a monoamine oxidase inhibitor; dothiepin, a tricyclic antidepressant; and mirtazapine, a noradrenergic and specific serotonergic antidepressant (Stevinson et al., 1999).

Mechanism of Action

It is unknown which constituent is responsible for the antidepressant effects. Hyperforin inhibits the uptake of serotonin, dopamine, noradrenaline, gamma-aminobutyric acid, and L-glutamate (Chatterjee et al., 1998).

Dosage

Capsules: 300 to 900 mg daily. Small children should receive a total of 300 mg daily, large children 600 mg daily, and adolescents the full adult dose (Bloomfield, Nordfors, and McWilliams, 1996). To determine effectiveness, the treatment period should last 4 to 6 weeks. Standardize to a hypericin content of 0.3 percent (Lenoir et al., 1999); some forms are standardized to 5 percent hyperforin (McCaleb et al., 2000).

Tincture: 20 to 30 drops three times daily (McCaleb et al., 2000).

Herbal oil: Massage oil into skin for tennis elbow, sprains, and strains.

Side Effects

Two cases of photosensitivity at high doses have been documented in humans. Larger-than-normal doses of St. John's wort have been known to cause dermatitis of the skin and inflammation of the mucous membranes after exposure to sunlight.

Contraindications

• Do not give St. John's wort to patients with chronic or severe depression.

Herb-Drug Interactions

St. John's wort should not be given with selective serotonin reuptake inhibitors (Lantz et al., 1999), nonsedating antihistamines, oral contraceptives, anti-retrovirals, anti-epileptics, calcium channel blockers, cyclosporine, chemotherapeutics, macrolide antibiotics, or antifungals (Roby et al., 2000). It may interfere with the metabolism of drugs used by AIDS patients (Piscitelli et al., 2000) and heart transplant patients (Ruschitzka et al., 2000). Do not give St. John's wort with any other antidepressant. After discontinuing a previous antidepressant, allow 2 weeks before starting St. John's wort, and taper the dosage.

Pregnancy and Breast-Feeding

No restrictions are known.

 # SUMMARY OF STUDIES

Schrader (2000). A randomized, controlled, 6-week German study of 242 outpatients compared St. John's wort to fluoxetine (Prozac). Of those, 114 patients took 20 mg of fluoxetine b.i.d. and 128 patients took Ze 117 hypericum extract tablet (Zeller, Switzerland) at 250 mg b.i.d. Results: St. John's wort had far superior safety and fewer, milder side effects than fluoxetine. The only side effect of St. John's wort was mild gastrointestinal upset.

Linde & Mulrow (1999). This meta-analysis included 27 random trials of 2291 participants. Results: There is evidence that extracts of hypericum are more effective than placebo for the treatment of mild to moderately severe depressive disorders.

Harrer & Schulz (1994). This report used 25 controlled clinical studies with 1592 subjects who took

300 to 900 mg for 2 to 6 weeks. Results: Hypericum was effective in the treatment of patients with mild to moderate depression. Studies indicate a high degree of efficacy and tolerability.

Sommer & Harrer (1994). This placebo-controlled, double-blind study included 89 subjects taking 300 mg t.i.d. for 4 weeks. Results: differences between active and placebo groups were statistically significant after 2 and 4 weeks; 67 percent of the active group responded to treatment, whereas 28 percent responded to the placebo.

Hubner & Kirste (2001). In a multicenter surveillance study, 101 children under 12 years old treated for 4 to 6 weeks with *Hypericum perforatum* at doses ranging from 300 to 1800 per day. Results showed that St. John's wort was safe and effective in treating mild depression and was without side effects.

REFERENCES

Bloomfield, H., Nordfors, M., & McWilliams, P. (1996). *Hypericum and depression.* CA: Prelude. Website at www.hypericum.com

Blumenthal, M., Goldberg, A., & Brinckmann, J. (Eds.). (2000). *Herbal medicine expanded Commission E monographs.* Austin, TX: American Botanical Council; Newton, MA: Integrative Medicine Communications.

Chatterjee, S., Bhattacharya, S., Wonnemann, M., et al. (1998). Hyperforin as a possible antidepressant component of *Hypericum* extracts. *Life Sciences, 63*(6), 499–510.

Harrer, G., & Schulz, V. (1994). Clinical investigation of the antidepressant effectiveness of hypericum. *Journal of Geriatric Psychiatry and Neurology, 7,* S6–S8.

Hubner, W. D., & Kirste, T. (2001). Experience with St. John's wort (*Hypericum perforatum*) in children under 12 years with symptoms of depression and psychovegetative disturbances. *Phytotherapy Research, 15*(4), 367–370.

Lantz, M., Buchalter, E., & Giambanco, V. (1999). St. John's wort and antidepressant drug interactions in the elderly. *Journal of Geriatric Psychiatry and Neurology, 12,* 7–10.

Lenoir, S., Degenring, F., & Saller, R.(1999). A double-blind randomized trial to investigate three different concentrations of a standardized fresh plant extract obtained from the shoot tips of H*ypericum perforatum* L. *Phytomedicine, 6*(3), 141–146.

Linde, K., & Mulrow, C. (1999). St. John's wort for depression. In *The Cochrane Library,* Issue 4, 1998. Oxford. Cited in *The integrative medicine consult* (February 1, 1999).

McCaleb, R., Leigh, E., & Morien, K. (2000). *The Encyclopedia of Popular Herbs.* Roseville, CA: Prima Publishing.

Murray, M. (1995). *The Healing Power of Herbs* (pp. 294–301). Roseville, CA: Prima Publishing.

Piscitelli, S. C., Burstein, A. H., Chai, H. D., Alfaro, R. M., & Falloon, J. (2000). Indinavir concentrations and St. John's wort. *The Lancet, 355,* 547–548.

Roby, C. A., Anderson, G. D., Kantor, E., Dryer,D. A., & Burstein, A. H. (2000). St. John's wort: Effect on CYP3A4 activity. *Clinical Pharmacology and Therapeutics, 67,* 451–457.

Ruschitzka, F., Meier, P. J., Turina, M., Luscher, T. F., & Noll, G. Acute heart transplant rejection due to St. John's wort. *The Lancet, 355,* 548–549.

Schrader, E. (2000). Equivalence of a St. John's wort extract (Ze 117) and fluoxetine: a randomized, controlled study in mild-moderate depression. *International Clinical Psychopharmacology, 15*(2), 61–68.

Shelton, R., et al. (2001). Effectiveness of St. John's wort in major depression. *Journal of the American Medical Association, 285,* 1978–1986.

Sommer, H., & Harrer, G. (1994). Placebo-controlled double-blind study examining the effectiveness of an *hypericum* preparation in 105 mildly depressed patients. *Journal of Geriatric Psychiatry and Neurology, 7,* S9–S11.

Stevinson, C., & Ernst, E.(1999). Safety of *Hypericum* in patients with depression: a comparison with conventional antidepressants. *CNS Drugs, 11*(2), 125–132.

NOTES

NOTES

ST. JOHN'S WORT
(Hypericum perforatum)

Historical Uses

St. John's wort was used by the ancient Greeks for sciatica and nervous disorders. It has also been used as a popular folk remedy for neuralgias, sciatica, burns or bruises involving nerve damage, sprains, emotional disorders, wounds, and tennis elbow.

Growth

This plant grows in fields and on roadsides throughout the United States. It reaches about 1 to 3 feet in height, and its yellow flowers bloom from June to September.

Parts Used

• Aerial (above-ground) parts

Medical Uses

St. John's wort is taken orally for mild to moderate depression, not for severe depression or bipolar disorder. It can be used externally for tennis elbow, sprains, and strains.

Dosage

Capsules: 300 to 900 mg daily. Small children should receive a total of 300 mg daily, large children 600 mg daily, and adolescents the full adult dose. To determine effectiveness, the treatment period should last 4 to 6 weeks. It is usually standardized to a hypericin content of 0.3 percent; some forms are standardized to 5 percent hyperforin.

Tincture: 20 to 30 drops three times daily.

Herbal oil: Massage oil into skin for tennis elbow, sprains, and strains.

Warnings

• St. John's wort may cause a rash in fair-skinned people.
• Larger-than-normal doses of St. John's wort may cause skin irritation and inflammation of the mucous membranes with exposure to sunlight.
• Don't take St. John's wort if you have chronic or severe depression.
• Consult with your health-care practitioner before using St. John's wort if you take any prescription medications, especially antidepressants, over-the-counter antihist-

amines for cold and allergy symptoms, oral birth control pills, HIV or AIDS medications, seizure medications, some heart medications, some antibiotics, and chemotherapy agents.

RECIPES

MASSAGE OIL (HERBAL OIL INFUSION) FOR STRAINS AND SPRAINS

Pick the buds of St. Johns' wort when the leaves are dotted with red spots (your fingers will turn red as you pick them). Place the buds (either dry or wilted) gently into a container and cover with extra virgin olive oil (thicker than other oils), or almond, sunflower, or safflower oil. Make sure that none of the plant parts extend above the oil or the oil will become moldy. Shake the jar daily. Place in a sunny area and in about 2 weeks the oil will turn red. Strain the herb into a dark bottle and use the oil all winter for any type of strain, sprain, backache, or sports injury.

SAW PALMETTO
(Serenoa repens)

Historical Uses

Saw palmetto berries were used by Native Americans for food and for medicinal effects. Traditional use has been as a tonic for men.

Growth

Saw palmetto is a short palm tree with sharp leaves that flourishes in the southern United States. Berries appear at the end of the summer months, and they turn a purplish black color. Saw palmetto is difficult to cultivate.

Part Used

• Fruit (berries)

Major Chemical Compounds

• Free fatty acids
• Sitosterols

Clinical Uses

Saw palmetto is used for benign prostatic hyperplasia (BPH), stages I and II.

Mechanism of Action

Saw palmetto inhibits the conversion of testosterone to dihydrotestosterone (as does finasteride [Proscar], a drug prescribed for treating BPH). It also speeds the breakdown and elimination of other hormones that are responsible for prostate enlargement. It reduces inflammation and fluid accumulation by a nonhormonal mechanism (Overmyer, 1999) that does not affect serum prostate-specific antigen (PSA) levels, thereby limiting the risk that treatment could mask the development of prostate cancer (Braeckman, 1994; Overmyer, 1999). Saw palmetto also has androgenic and antiprostatitic activity (Duke, 2000).

Dosage

Standardized extract: 160 mg twice daily or 320 mg of standardized extract daily for BPH. It is standardized to 85 to 95 percent fatty acids and sterols. Results are usually noted in 30 days. Continue for 4 to 6 months with follow-up by primary care

243

provider if medication needs to continue on a long-term basis. Saw palmetto does not interfere with results of PSA tests (McCaleb et al., 2000).

Side Effects

Saw palmetto may cause mild stomach upset.

Contraindications

• Saw palmetto is not recommended for patients with bacterial prostatitis.

Herb-Drug Interactions

Saw palmetto may decrease iron absorption.

Pregnancy and Breast-Feeding

Saw palmetto is safe when used appropriately.

Pediatric Patients

Saw palmetto is not recommended for children.

SUMMARY OF STUDIES

Marks et al. (2000). In this controlled, 6-month trial (an American study), 44 subjects took a blend of saw palmetto extract, nettle root extract, and pumpkin seed oil (Nutrilite, product of Amway) for BPH symptoms Results: symptoms improved, but not to a statistically significant degree. The saw palmetto combination product slowed the growth of prostate tissue via a nonhormonal mechanism without affecting serum PSA levels.

Overmyer (1999). A randomized, double-blind, placebo-controlled clinical trial used saw palmetto extract for 44 men with BPH. Results: Saw palmetto was beneficial in reducing swelling of prostate tissues by an unidentified nonhormonal mechanism in patients with BPH without affecting PSA levels.

Wilt et al. (1998). This meta-analysis of 18 studies (16 double-blind, placebo-controlled trials lasting 30 days to 48 weeks) involved 2939 men who had symptomatic BPH. Results: Compared to placebo, saw palmetto was associated with a lower frequency of nighttime urination and an improvement in peak urine flow. When saw palmetto was compared to Proscar, saw palmetto subjects said that adverse effects were mild and infrequent and erectile dysfunction was lower. Side effects of saw palmetto were 1.1 percent and those of Proscar were 4.9 percent.

Braeckman (1994). An uncontrolled, open trial of 505 patients with BPH lasted for 3 months. Patients were given 160 mg of saw palmetto b.i.d. for 3 months. After 90 days of treatment, 88 percent of patients and doctors said that therapy was effective. Side effects were reported in 5 percent of patients.

Romics et al. (1993). An uncontrolled clinical trial of 42 subjects lasted 12 months. Patients were given 160 mg of saw palmetto for 12 months. Results: Symptoms improved without side effects.

DiSilverio et al. (1992). In this double-blind, placebo-controlled study, 35 patients with BPH were randomized into two groups. Results: Saw palmetto has more of an antiestrogenic effect and less of an antiandrogenic effect.

Smith et al. (1986). This double-blind comparison involved Permixon (trade name of saw palmetto) 160 mg q.d. Results: Saw palmetto produced significant improvement in flow rate and BPH symptoms compared to placebo results.

Champault, G. (1984). This double-blind, placebo-controlled study included 94 patients with BPH for 30 days. Permixon at 80 mg b.i.d. was well tolerated with fewer side effects. Side effects were minor (e.g., headache). There were no changes in laboratory test results.

Schneider, H., Masuhr, T., (1995). A prospective, longitudinal, observational study of 2080 patients with BPH used saw palmetto. Results: Symptomatic. improvement was reported in 86 percent of subjects and improved quality of life was reported by 80 percent. Among physicians, 87 percent reported efficacy as very good or good.

REFERENCES

Blumenthal, M., Goldberg, A., & Brinckmann, J. (Eds.). (2000). *Herbal medicine expanded Commission E monographs* (pp. 335–340). Austin, TX: American Botanical Council; Newton, MA: Integrative Medicine Communications.

Braeckman, J. (1994). The extract of *Serenoa repens* in the treatment of BPH: A multicenter open study. *Current Therapeutic Research, 55,* 776–785.

Brown, D. (1995). *An introduction to phytotherapy: The medical uses of 8 common herbs.* Connecticut: Keats.

Champault, G., Patel, J., & Bonnard, A. (1984). A double blind trial of an extract of the plant *Serenoa repens* in BPH. *British Journal of Clinical Pharmacology, 18,* 461–462.

DiSilverio, F., et al. (1992). Evidence that *Serenoa repens* extract displays an antiestrogenic activity in prostatic tissue of BPH. *European Urology, 21,* 309–314.

Duke, J. (2000) Phytochemical and Ethnobotanical Database at the Agricultural Research Services.

Marks, L., et al. (2000). Effects of a saw palmetto herbal blend in men with symptomatic benign prostatic hyperplasia. *Journal of Urology, 163*(5), 1451–1456.

McCaleb, R. (March 1996). Herbal help for prostate problems. *Herbs for Health,* 27–28.

McGuffin, M., Hobbs, C., Upton, R., & Goldberg, A. (1997). *Botanical safety handbook* (p, 107). Boca Raton, FL: CRC Press.

Miller, L. (1998). Herbal medicinals: Selected clinical considerations focusing on known or potential drug-herb interactions. *Archives of Internal Medicine, 158,* 2200–2211. Cited in Vickers & Zollman (1999). Herbal medicine. *British Medical Journal, 319,* 1050–1053.

Overmyer, M. (1999). Saw palmetto shown to shrink prostatic epithelium. *Urology Times, 27*(6), 1, 42.

Romics, I., Schmitz, H., & Frang, D. (1993). Experience in treating benign prostatic hypertrophy with *Sabal serrulata* for one year. *International Urology and Nephrology, 25,* 565–569.

Schneider, H., & Masuhr, T. (1995). Treatment of benign prostatic hyperplasia: Results of a surveillance study in the practices of urological specialists using a combined plant-based preparation. *Fortschritte der Medizin, 113:*37–40.

Smith, H., Memon, A., Smart, C., & Dewbury, K.(1986).The value of Permixon in BPH. *British Journal of Urology, 58,* 36–40.

Wilt, T. J., et al (1998). Saw palmetto extracts for treatment of benign prostatic hyperplasia. *Journal of the American Medical Association, 158*(18), 1604–1609.

NOTES

SAW PALMETTO
(Serenoa repens)

Historical Uses

Saw palmetto berries were used by Native Americans for food and for medicinal effects. Traditional use has been as a tonic for men.

Growth

Saw palmetto is a short palm tree with sharp leaves that flourishes in the southern United States. Berries appear at the end of the summer months, and they turn a purplish black color. Saw palmetto is difficult to cultivate.

Part Used

- Fruit (berries)

Medical Uses

Saw palmetto is used for benign prostatic hyperplasia (BPH), stages I and II.

Dosage

Standardized extract: 160 mg twice daily or 320 mg of standardized extract daily for BPH. It is standardized to 85 to 95 percent fatty acids and sterols. Results are usually noted in 30 days. Continue for 4 to 6 months with follow-up by primary care provider if medication needs to continue on a long-term basis. Saw palmetto does not interfere with results of the prostate-specific antigen test.

Warnings

- Saw palmetto may cause mild stomach upset.
- Don't take saw palmetto if you have bacterial prostatitis.
- This herb may decrease iron absorption.
- Saw palmetto is safe during pregnancy and breast-feeding when used appropriately.
- It isn't recommended for children.

SHIITAKE MUSHROOM
(Lentinus edodes)

Historical Uses

The most common edible mushroom in the world, the shiitake mushroom is also known as the black forest mushroom, the Chinese mushroom, and the king of mushrooms. In China, shiitake mushrooms have been eaten medicinally for centuries to boost the immune system (McCaleb et al., 2000).

Growth

Shiitake mushrooms grow in Japan on fallen shiia trees. This mushroom is native to China, Japan, and other parts of Asia, but not to the United States.

Parts Used

- Fruiting body
- Mycelium

Major Chemical Compounds

- Polysaccharides

Clinical Uses

Shiitake mushroom is used for candidiasis, colds, allergies, and heart disease. It is active against lung cancer and melanoma (Ladanyi et al., 1993), and it has hypolipidemic and antithrombotic effects (Mizuno, 1995).

Mechanism of Action

This mushroom increases the production and ability of natural killer cells and macrophages to destroy tumor cells (Ladanyi et al., 1993). Polysaccharides bind to specialized receptor sites on macrophages and natural killer cells, thereby sending out chemical signals to fight off infection (Roundtree, 2000).

Dosage

Fresh mushrooms: 3 to 4 mushrooms daily.

Capsules: 400 mg taken 1 to 5 times daily.

Tincture: One dropperful 2 to 3 times daily (McCaleb et al., 2000).

Vitamin C may help in the absorption of polysaccharides (McCaleb et al., 2000).

Side Effects

Shiitake mushroom may cause skin rash or stomach upset (McCaleb et al., 2000).

Contraindications

- Ingestion of more than 4 grams of shiitake powder daily for 10 weeks may cause eosinophilia (Levy, 1998).
- Do not give shiitake mushroom to patients with eosinophilia (*Natural Medicine*, 2000).

Herb-Drug Interactions

None are known.

Pregnancy and Breast-Feeding

No restrictions are known (McGuffin et al., 1997).

SUMMARY OF STUDIES

Limited clinical research on humans is available.

Chang (1996). In this review, edible mushrooms such as shiitake mushrooms were found to contain functional "nutraceutical" or medicinal properties that benefit the immune system, lower lipids, and have antitumor properties without toxic effecs.

REFERENCES

Chang, R. (1996). Functional properties of edible mushrooms. *Nutrition Review, 54*(11, Pt. 2), S91–S93.

Hobbs, C. (January/February 2000). Cancer-fighting mushrooms. *Herbs for Health,* 59–60.

Ladanyi, A., Timar, J., & Lapis, K. (1993). Effect of Lentinan on macrophage cytoxicity against metastatic tumor cells. *Cancer Immunology, Immunotherapy, 36*, 123–6.[Medline]

Levy, A. M., Kita, H., Phillips, S. F., Schnade, P. A., Dyer, P. D., Gleich, G. J., & Dubravec, V. A. (1998). Eosinophilia and gastrointestinal symptoms after ingestion of shiitake mushrooms. *Journal of Allergy and Clinical Immunology, 101*(5), 613–620.

McCaleb, R., Leigh, E., & Morien, K. (2000). *The Encyclopedia of Popular Herbs.* Roseville, CA: Prima Publishing.

McGuffin, M., Hobbs, C., Upton, R., & Goldberg, A. (1997). *Botanical Safety Handbook.* Boca Raton, FL: CRC Press.

Mizuno, T. (1995). *Shiitake Lentinus edodes:* Functional properties for medicinal and food purposes. *Food Rev Int., 11,* 111–128.

Natural Medicines Comprehensive Database. (2000). *Pharmacist's Letter and Prescriber's Letter.* Therapeutic Research Faculty.

Roundtree, R. (November/December 2000). Immune suppressants and herbal medicines. *Herbs for Health,* 26–27.

NOTES

SHIITAKE MUSHROOM
(Lentinus edodes)

Historical Uses

The most common edible mushroom in the world, the shiitake mushroom is also known as the black forest mushroom, the Chinese mushroom, and the king of mushrooms. In China, shiitake mushrooms have been eaten medicinally for centuries to boost the immune system.

Growth

Shiitake mushrooms grow in Japan on fallen shiia trees. This mushroom is native to China, Japan, and other parts of Asia, but not to the United States.

Parts Used
- Fruiting body
- Mycelium

Major Chemical Compounds
- Polysaccharides

This mushroom is rich in vitamins D, B_2, and B_{12}. It contains about 2.5 percent protein.

Medical Uses

Shiitake mushroom is used for candidiasis (yeast infections), colds, allergies, and heart disease.

Dosage

Fresh mushrooms: 3 to 4 mushrooms daily.

Capsules: 400 mg taken 1 to 5 times daily.

Tincture: One dropperful 2 to 3 times daily.

Vitamin C may help in the absorption of polysaccharides.

Warnings
- Shiitake mushrooms may cause skin rash and stomach upset.
- Ingestion of more than 4 grams of shiitake powder daily for 10 weeks may cause serious side effects. Talk to your health-care practitioner if you have a blood disorder.
- Shiitake mushroom is safe for pregnant and breast-feeding women when consumed in food amounts.

RECIPES

Buy fresh or dried mushrooms and add them to soups, stir-fries, or side dishes. Soak dried mushrooms in water for a few hours or overnight before adding them to food.

SHIITAKE MUSHROOMS AND BROWN RICE

Start the brown rice before you start the mushrooms. (Although brown rice takes a little longer than white rice [about 45 minutes], it is well worth the wait because it has more vitamins, minerals, and flavor). Add fresh or rehydrated shiitake mushrooms (whole or sliced) to a sauté pan to which you've also added olive oil. Add a few onions and garlic, and then add the cooked rice.

MEDICINAL MUSHROOM SOUP

Make a soup out of 50 grams of fresh or dried shiitake mushrooms, vegetables, grains, and beans. This combination offers a wonderful way to boost the immune system and reduce the side effects of chemotherapy and radiation therapy.

INFECTION BUSTER

Add 1 to 3 shiitake mushrooms per person (including children) to stir-fries, vegetables, or chicken soup to help ward off winter illnesses.

SLIPPERY ELM
(Ulmus rubra)

Historical Uses

Native Americans and early settlers used slippery elm bark for coughs, sore throats, and bronchitis. Native Americans also used slippery elm bark during labor and for poultices for burns and mastitis (Weiss, 1985). In folklore, slippery elm bark was used to make a nutritive broth for children and elderly people (Foster and Duke, 1990).

Growth

The red elm tree grows in the central and northern United States. It prefers to grow in woods, particularly on the banks of streams, but it will also grow in poor soil. When the tree is 10 years old, its bark can be used for its medicinal effects.

Part Used

• Inner bark

Major Chemical Compounds

• Mucilage
• Tannin

Clinical Uses

Slippery elm bark is used for irritations of the mucous membranes, coughs, sore throats, and diarrhea. It is also used to help stop *Candida* overgrowth.

Mechanism of Action

Mucilage restores the normal mucous coating of irritated tissues.

Dosage

Tea: For acute conditions, mix 1 teaspoon of slippery elm bark powder and 1 teaspoon of sugar in 2 cups of boiling water and let sit for 10 minutes. Season with cinnamon or nutmeg. Drink 1 to 2 cups daily.

Lozenges: Let one lozenge dissolve in the mouth every 4 hours as needed.

253

Side Effects

None are known.

Contraindications

• None are known.

Herb-Drug Interactions

None are known.

Pregnancy and Breast-Feeding

No restrictions are known (McGuffin et al., 1997).

SUMMARY OF STUDIES

No recent clinical studies in humans are available.

REFERENCES

Foster, S., & Duke, J. (1990). *Eastern/central medicinal plants* (p. 294). New York: Houghton Mifflin.

McGuffin, M., Hobbs, C., Upton, R., & Goldberg, A. (1997). *Botanical safety handbook*. Boca Raton, FL: CRC Press.

NOTES

SLIPPERY ELM
(Ulmus rubra)

Historical Uses

Native Americans and early settlers used slippery elm bark for coughs, sore throats, and bronchitis. Native Americans also used slippery elm bark during labor and for poultices for burns and mastitis. In folklore, slippery elm bark was used to make a nutritive broth for children and elderly people.

Growth

The red elm tree grows in the central and northern United States. It prefers to grow in woods, particularly on the banks of streams, but it will also grow in poor soil. When the tree is 10 years old, its bark can be used for its medicinal effects.

Part Used

• Inner bark

Medical Uses

Slippery elm bark is used for irritations of the mucous membranes, coughs, sore throats, and diarrhea. It is also used to help stop yeast infections.

Dosage

Tea: For acute conditions, mix 1 teaspoon of slippery elm bark powder and 1 teaspoon of sugar in 2 cups of boiling water and let sit for 10 minutes. Season with cinnamon or nutmeg. Drink 1 to 2 cups daily.

Lozenges: Let one lozenge dissove in your mouth every 4 hours as needed.

Warnings

• None are known.

RECIPES

SLIPPERY ELM BARK LEMONADE FOR COLDS AND BRONCHITIS

Mix 1 tablespoon of slippery elm bark powder with cold water to make a paste. Add 1 pint of boiling water and stir in the juice of half a lemon. Add honey to taste.

SOY

(Glycine max)

Historical Uses

In China, soy is valued highly and has been called one of the five sacred grains.

Growth

Soy is a subtropical plant that is now cultivated in temperate regions. The plant grows from 1 to 5 feet tall.

Part Used

• Seed (soybean)

Major Chemical Compounds

• Genistein, a major isoflavone in soy and a weak estrogen
• Daidzein, another isoflavone

Clinical Uses

Soy is used to treat high cholesterol (Anderson et al., 1995), diabetes mellitus (Holt et al., 1996), and menopausal symptoms and is also used for its anticancer effects (Craig, 1997) and prevention of osteoporosis (Potter et al., 1998; Arjmandi et al., 1998; Ramsey et al., 1999). Labels approved by the Food and Drug Administration state that soy may help lower cholesterol levels and reduce the risk of heart disease. Soy is approved by the German Commission E for mild hypercholesterolemia (Blumenthal et al., 2000).

Soy products containing isoflavones may provide a viable alternative to hormones for maintaining bone density and protecting against cardiovascular diseases, especially for postmenopausal women who choose to not take hormone replacement therapy. Japanese people consume an average of 7 to 10 grams of soy protein daily and about 30 to 50 mg of isoflavones daily. Soy may have implications for breast cancer prevention (Lu et al., 2001).

Mechanism of Action

The mechanism of action is unknown at this time, although we know that soy may have anticancer properties (Craig, 1997). It may protect against breast cancer by interfering with estradiol (acting as an anti-estrogen). Phytoestrogens, like isoflavones, have both estrogenic and anti-estrogenic effects (Ramsey et al., 1999). If phytoestrogens compete with natural estrogen to bind with body's estrogen receptors, they may decrease the receptors' ability to pick up estradiol in premenopausal women. In postmenopausal women, who have little of their own estradiol, phytoestrogens could have a small estrogenic effect (Ramsey et al., 1999).

Isoflavones enhance bone formation (Arjmandi et al., 1998). The mechanism of action of isoflavones is different from that of human estrogen (Arjmandi et al., 1998). The degree to which soy consumption decreases low-density lipoprotein levels is similar to that seen with hormone replacement therapy (Hulley et al., (1998).

Dosage

It is estimated that 200 mg of isoflavones are equal to about 0.3 mg of Premarin. The average dosage of Premarin is 0.625 mg daily (Hudson, 2000).

Isoflavones or soy protein: 40 to 100 mg of isoflavones or 30 to 50 grams of soy protein daily. Cholesterol-lowering benefits may occur with 25 grams (or 2 to 4 servings of soy foods) daily. For relief of hot flashes and maintenance of bone density, 40 to 60 grams daily may be needed (Natural Medicines, 2000). Do not exceed 100 mg per day of isoflavone supplements because the effect of large supplemental doses over long periods is unknown (Holt, 1997). For soy to be absorbed properly, healthy bacteria (acidophilus) are needed in the digestive tract (McCaleb et al., 2000).

Food sources: The more processed the soybean, the lower its nutritional value. Soybeans contain the most isoflavones (and about 80 mg of calcium per ½ cup), whereas soy oil and soy sauce have virtually none.

Soy milk: Soy milk contains the same amount of protein as cow's milk, one-third the fat of cow's milk, fewer calories than cow's milk, no cholesterol, many B vitamins, and 15 times as much iron, although cow's milk is higher in calcium (Knight, 2000; McCaleb et al., 2000; Ramsey et al., 1999). It can be drunk by the glass and used in recipes as a substitute for cow's milk. Soy milk contains about 10 grams of protein, 20 mg of isoflavones, and 250 to 300 mg of calcium (fortified) per cup. It is made by grinding soybeans, mixing them with water, boiling and filtering the liquid, and sweetening it with vanilla, chocolate, or carob.

Tofu: Tofu is curdled soy milk that is drained and pressed. Its firmness depends on the amount of whey it contains. Extra-firm tofu has the most protein and is great in stir-fry dishes. Firm tofu can be used in lasagnas. Soft tofu can be used for desserts or puddings. Tofu contains 15 grams of protein, 40 mg of isoflavones, and about 130 mg of calcium per ½ cup.

Textured soy protein: This form of soy is similar to ground beef or turkey and can be used in chili, lasagna, or tacos. It contains about 22 grams of protein and 170 mg of calcium per cup.

Tempeh: This form of soy is like a soybean cake. It can be baked, grilled, or microwaved. It is high in fiber and contains no cholesterol. It contains about 15 grams of protein, 60 mg of isoflavones, and 77 mg of calcium per ½ cup.

Soy powder: This form of soy is high in protein, B vitamins, and iron. It can be added to fruit shakes or milkshakes.

Side Effects

Soy, especially soy protein powder, may cause bloating, nausea, and constipation.

Contraindications

• Soy is contraindicated in patients who are allergic to it.
• Soybeans should not be eaten raw.

Herb-Drug Interactions

None are known.

Pregnancy and Breast-Feeding

No restrictions are known if soy is consumed as a food. Isoflavone supplements are not recommended during pregnancy (Holt, 1997).

Pediatric Patients

Isoflavone supplements are not recommended in children(Holt, 1997).

 # SUMMARY OF STUDIES

The National Institutes of Health are currently studying soy isoflavones and their effects in preventing breast, prostate, colon, and lung cancer.

Potter et al. (1998). This double-blind study of postmenopausal women looked at the effects of soy isoflavones on bone density over a 6-month period. One group of women consumed 40 grams of non-soy protein daily; the other consumed soy-based protein with high levels of isoflavones (2.25 mg of isoflavones per gram of protein). Results: Spinal bone density increased in the group that consumed high levels of isoflavones.

Anderson et al. (1995). This meta-analysis included 38 controlled trials of soy and serum lipids. Results: Soy protein at about 47 grams daily decreased total cholesterol levels by 9.3 percent, low-density lipoprotein levels by 12.9 percent, and triglyceride levels by 10.5 percent.

Ho et al. (2001). In this longitudinal study, 132 women aged 30 to 40 years were followed for 3 years. Soy intake had a significant effect on the maintenance of spinal bone mineral density in this age group.

REFERENCES

Anderson, J., Johnstone, B., & Cook-Newall, M. (1995). Meta-analysis of the effects of soy protein intake on serum lipids. *New England Journal of Medicine, 333,* 276–282.

Arjmandi, B., Birnbaum, R., Goyal, N., et al. (1998). Bone-sparing effect of soy protein in ovarian hormone-deficient rats is related to its isoflavone content. *American Journal of Clinical Nutrition, 68*(6 Suppl), 1364S–1368S.

Arjmandi, B., Getlinger, M., Goyal, N., Alekel, L., Hasler, C. M., Juma, S., Drum, M. L., Hollis, B. U., & Kukreja, S. C. (1998). Role of soy protein with normal or reduced isoflavone content in reversing bone loss induced by ovarian deficiency in rats. *American Journal of Clinical Nutrition, 68,* 1358S–1363S.

Blumenthal, M., Goldberg, A., & Brinckmann, J. (Eds.). (2000). *Herbal medicine expanded Commission E monographs.* Austin, TX: American Botanical Council; Newton, MA: Integrative Medicine Communications.

Craig, W. (1997). Phytochemicals: Guardians of our health. *Journal of the American Diet Association, 10* (Suppl 2), S199–204.

Ho, S. C., Chan, S. G., Yi, Q., Wong, E., & Leung, P. C. (2001). Soy intake and the maintenance of peak bone mass in Hong Kong Chinese women. *Journal of Bone and Mineral Research, 16*(7), 1363–1369.

Holt, S. (1997). Phytoestrogens for a healthier menopause. *Alternative and Complementary Therapies, 3*(3), 187–193.

Holt, S., Muntyan, I., & Likver, L. (1996). Soya-based diets for diabetes mellitus. *Alternative and Complementary Therapies, 2*(2), 79–82.

Hulley, S., Grady, D., Bush, T., Furberg, C., Herrington, D., Riggs, B., & Vittinghoff, E. (1998). Randomized trial of estrogen plus progestin for secondary prevention of coronary heart disease in postmenopausal women. *Journal of the American Medical Association, 280,* 605–613.

Knight, J. (November/December 2000). Soy meets world. *Herbs for Health,* 39–44.

Lu, L. J., Anderson, K. E., Grady, J. J., & Nagamani, M. (2001). Effects of an isoflavone-free soy diet on ovarian hormones in premenopausal women. *The Journal of Clinical Endocrinology and Metabolism, 86*(7), 3045–3052.

McCaleb, R., Leigh, E., & Morien, K. (2000). *The Encyclopedia of Popular Herbs.* Roseville, CA: Prima Publishing.

Potter, S., Baum, J., Teng, H., Stillman, R., Shay, N., & Erdman, J., Jr. (1998). Soy protein and isoflavones: Their effects on blood lipids and bone density in post-menopausal women. *American Journal of Clinical Nutrition, 68*(6 Suppl), 1375S–1379S.

Natural Medicines Comprehensive Database. (2000). *Pharmacist's Letter and Prescriber's Letter.* (Soy supplements, p. 58).Therapeutic Research Faculty.

Ramsey, L., Ross, B., & Fischer, R. (May 1999). Management of menopause. *Advance for Nurse Practitioners,* 27–30.

NOTES

SOY
(Glycine max)

Historical Uses

In China, soy is valued highly and has been called one of the five sacred grains.

Growth

Soy is a subtropical plant that is now cultivated in temperate regions. The plant grows from 1 to 5 feet tall.

Part Used

• Seed (soybean)

Medical Uses

Soy is used for high cholesterol, diabetes mellitus, and menopausal symptoms and is also used for its anticancer effects and prevention of osteoporosis. Labels approved by the Food and Drug Administration state that soy may help lower cholesterol levels and reduce the risk of heart disease.

Dosage

It is estimated that 200 mg of isoflavones are equal to about 0.3 mg of Premarin. The average dosage of Premarin is 0.625 mg daily.

Isoflavones or soy protein: 40 to 100 mg of isoflavones or 30 to 50 grams of soy protein daily. Cholesterol-lowering benefits may occur with 25 grams (or 2 to 4 servings of soy foods) daily. Relief of hot flashes and maintenance of bone density may need 40 to 60 grams daily. Do not exceed 100 mg per day of isoflavone supplements because the effects of large supplemental doses over long periods is unknown (Holt, 1997). For soy to be absorbed properly, healthy bacteria (acidophilus) are needed in the digestive tract.

Food sources: The more processed the soybean, the lower its nutritional value. Soybeans contain the most isoflavones (and about 80 mg of calcium per 1/2 cup), whereas soy oil and soy sauce have virtually none.

Soy milk: In comparison to cow's milk, soy milk contains the same amount of protein, one-third the fat, fewer calories, no cholesterol, many B vitamins, and 15 times as much iron, although cow's milk is higher in calcium. Drink it by the glass, and use it in recipes as a substitute for cow's milk. Soy milk contains about 10 grams of protein, 20 mg of isoflavones, and 250 to 300 mg of calcium (fortified) per cup. It is made by grinding soybeans, mixing them with water, boiling and filtering the liquid, and sweetening it with vanilla, chocolate, or carob.

Tofu: Tofu is curdled soy milk that is drained and pressed. Its firmness depends on the amount of whey it contains. Extra-firm tofu has the most protein and is great in stir-fry dishes. Firm tofu can be used in lasagnas. Soft tofu can be used for desserts or puddings. Tofu contains 15 grams of protein, 40 mg of isoflavones, and about 130 mg of calcium per 1/2 cup.

Textured soy protein: This form of soy is similar to ground beef or turkey and can be used in chili, lasagna, or tacos. It contains about 22 grams of protein and 170 mg of calcium per cup.

Tempeh: This form of soy is like a soybean cake. It can be baked, grilled, or microwaved. It is high in fiber and contains no cholesterol. It contains about 15 grams of protein, 60 mg of isoflavones, and 77 mg of calcium per 1/2 cup.

Soy powder: This form of soy is high in protein, B vitamins, and iron. It can be added to fruit shakes or milkshakes.

Warnings

- Don't eat raw soybeans.
- Soy may cause allergic reactions.
- Soy, especially soy protein powder, may cause bloating, nausea, and constipation.
- No restrictions are known for pregnant and breast-feeding women if soy is consumed as a food.
- Isoflavone supplements aren't recommended for children or pregnant women.

TEA TREE OIL
(Melaleuca alternifolia)

Historical Uses

In folklore, tea tree oil has been used for its antiseptic effects and to treat fungal infections and coughs. During World War II, 1 percent tea tree oil was used to prevent skin injuries in munitions factory workers in Australia (Tyler, 1993).

Growth

A tea tree is a small tree or shrub with heads of stalkless yellow or purplish flowers (Lawless, 1997).

Part Used

• Leaves, extracted by steam or water distillation (Lawless, 1997).

Major Chemical Compounds

• Linalool
• Terpinolene
• Alpha-terpineol, made up of primarily monoterpenes and alcohols.

Clinical Uses

Tea tree oil has antibacterial properties (Carson et al.,1995) and antifungal properties (Buck et al., 1994). It also is used for acne (Bassett et al., 1990) and herpes simplex (Schnitzler et al., 2001).

Mechanism of Action

Major chemical compounds in tea tree oil are active against *Candida albicans* (Pena, 1962), trichophytons, *Staphylococcus aureus,* and *Trichomonas vaginalis* (Pena, 1962).

Dosage

Acne: Use a swab to apply directly to acne cysts twice daily. Avoid the eye area.

Onychomycosis: Use a swab to apply to fingernails or toenails twice daily. Avoid getting oil on the skin.

Side Effects

None are known.

Contraindications

• Tea tree oil should not be taken internally.

Pregnancy and Breast-Feeding

Tea tree oil is not for use during pregnancy.

SUMMARY OF STUDIES

Carson et al. (1995). This in vitro study showed that methicillin-resistant *Staphylococcus aureus* was susceptible to tea tree oil.

Buck et al. (1994). This double-blind, multicenter trial involving 117 patients with chronic toenail onychomycosis caused by *Trichophyton* compared pure tea tree oil with 1 percent clotrimazole solution. Results: tea tree oil compared favorably with clotrimazole over a 6-month time period.

Bassett et al. (1990). This 3-month, randomized clinical trial included 124 patients with mild to moderate acne who used either tea tree oil 5 percent or 5 percent benzoyl peroxide in water-based gel and lotion. Results: Both treatments significantly reduced the number of lesions. Tea tree oil took longer to act, but it caused less irritating side effects.

Pena (1962). In this study, patients applied tea tree oil 40 percent in 13 percent isopropyl alcohol on a tampon along with daily vaginal douches and office visits. Results: Tea tree oil was as effective as antitrichomonal suppositories. Vaginal candidiasis also resolved.

Ernst & Huntley (2000). In a review of randomized trials using tea tree oil, "evidence is promising for treatment of acne and fungal infection."

REFERENCES

Bassett, I., Pannowitz, D., & Barnetson, R. (1990). A comparative study of tea-tree oil versus benzoylperoxide in the treatment of acne. *Medical Journal of Australia, 153,* 455–458.

Buck, D., Nidorf, D., & Addino, J. (1994). Comparison of two topical preparations for the treatment of onychomycosis: *Melaleuca alternifolia* (tea tree) oil and clotrimazole. *Journal of Family Practice, 38,* 601–605.

Carson, C., Cookson, B., Farrelly, et al. (1995). Susceptibility of methicillin-resistant *Staphylococcus aureus* to the essential oil of *Melaleuca alternifolia. Journal of Antimicrobial Chemotherapy, 35,* 421–424.

Carson, C., & Riley, T. (1995). Antimicrobial activity of the major components of the essential oil of *Melaleuca alternifolia. Journal of Applied Bacteriology, 78,* 264–269.

Ernst, E., & Huntley, A. (2000). Tea tree oil: A systematic review of randomized clinical trials. *Forschende Komplementarmedizin und Klassische Naturheilkunde [Research in Complementary and Natural Classical Medicine], 7*(1), 17–20.

Lawless, J. (1997). *The complete illustrated guide to aromatherapy.* Boston: Element Books Limited.

Pena, E. (1962). *Melaleuca alternifolia* oil. *Obstetrics and Gynecology, 19,* 793–795.

Schnitzler, P., Schon, K., & Reichling, J. (2001). Antiviral activity of Australian tea tree oil and eucalyptus oil against herpes simplex virus in cell culture. *Pharmazie, 56*(4), 343–347.

Tyler, V. (1993). *The honest herbal.* Binghamton, NY: Pharmaceutical Products Press.

NOTES

NOTES

TEA TREE OIL
(Melaleuca alternifolia)

Historical Uses

In folklore, tea tree oil has been used for antiseptic effects and to treat fungal infections and coughs. During World War II, 1 percent tea tree oil was used to prevent skin injuries in munitions factory workers in Australia.

Growth

A tea tree is a small tree or shrub with heads of stalkless yellow or purplish flowers.

Part Used

• Leaves, extracted by steam or water distillation.

Medical Uses

Tea tree oil has antibacterial and antifungal properties. It is also used for acne.

Dosage

Acne: Use a swab to apply directly to acne cysts twice daily. Avoid the eye area.

Onychomycosis: Use a swab to apply to fingernails or toenails twice daily. Avoid getting oil on the skin.

Warnings

• Do not take tea tree oil internally.
• Do not use tea tree oil during pregnancy or when breast-feeding.
• Do not use tea tree oil near the eyes.

RECIPES

Tea tree oil can be used as a disinfectant for house cleaning. Add 50 drops of essential oil to your usual laundry detergent in the washing machine, or add it to a bucket of warm water for washing the floor.

TOMATO

(Lycopersicon esculentum)

Historical Uses

Historically, tomato was used medicinally for gout and rheumatism. The tomato has been consumed as a food in the U. S. for the past 80 years and today is the third most common vegetable eaten in the U. S. (Wood, 1999).

Growth

Tomato is a common commercial vegetable crop and is commonly grown in home vegetable gardens in the summer.

Part Used

- Fruit

Major Chemical Compounds

- Lycopene
- Sugar
- Fiber
- Flavonoids and other phytochemicals
- Vitamin C
- Vitamins A and B
- Potassium
- Phosphorus

Clinical Uses

Tomato has anticarcinogenic effects on prostate cancer.

Mechanism of Action

Lycopene fights cancer by neutralizing free-radical oxygen molecules before they can damage cells (Djuric & Powell, 2001).

Dosage

Tomatoes may be consumed fresh, in sauce, or as tomato juice.

To prevent prostate cancer: Four or more servings of tomato products each week, which translates to more than 6 mg of lycopene per daily (Giovannucci et al., 1995). Lycopene is higher in ketchup, tomato juice, tomato paste, tomato sauce, and cooked tomatoes than in fresh tomatoes. One cup of tomato juice contains about 23 mg of lycopene (*Natural Medicines, 2000*).

Tomatoes should not be cooked in aluminum or cast iron utensils; their acid binds with these metals and food will taste metallic.

Side Effects

None are known.

Contraindications

• The tomato leaf and vine may be unsafe to eat (*Natural Medicines*, 2000).

Herb-Drug Interactions

None are known.

Pregnancy and Breast-Feeding

No restrictions are known.

 # SUMMARY OF STUDIES

Giovannucci et al. (*1995*). This prospective cohort study included 48,000 men. Results: The risk of prostate cancer was inversely associated with the consumption of tomatoes.

REFERENCES

Brody, J (1985). *Jane Brody's good food book.* (p. 521). New York: W.W. Norton & Co.

Djuric, Z., & Powell, L. C. (2001). Antioxidant capacity of lycopene-containing foods. *International Journal of Food Sciences and Nutrition, 52*(2), 143–149.

Giovannucci, E., Ascherio, A., Rimm, E. B., et al. (1995). Intake of carotenoids and retinol in relation to risk of prostate cancer. *Journal of National Cancer Institute, 87,* 1767–1776.

Natural Medicines Comprehensive Database. (2000). *Pharmacist's Letter and Prescriber's Letter.* Therapeutic Research Faculty.

Wood, R. (1999). *The new whole foods encyclopedia.* New York: Penguin, p. 159.

NOTES

NOTES

TOMATO
⟨Lycopersicon esculentum⟩

Historical Uses

Historically, tomato was used medicinally for gout and rheumatism. The tomato has been consumed as a food in the U. S. for the past 80 years and today is the third most common vegetable eaten in the U. S.

Growth

Tomato is a common commercial vegetable crop and is commonly grown in home vegetable gardens in the summer.

Part Used

• Fruit

Clinical Uses

Tomato has anticarcinogenic effects on prostate cancer.

Dosage

To prevent prostate cancer: Four or more servings of tomato products each week, which translates to more than 6 mg of lycopene per daily. Lycopene is higher in ketchup, tomato juice, tomato paste, tomato sauce, and cooked tomatoes than in fresh tomatoes. One cup of tomato juice contains about 23 mg of lycopene.

Tomatoes should not be cooked in aluminum or cast iron; their acid binds with these metals and food will taste metallic.

Warnings

• Don't eat tomato leaves or vines; they may be unsafe to eat.

RECIPES

MIDDLE EASTERN RATATOUILLE

Make this dish when tomatoes are plentiful and freeze it for use throughout the year. The recipe is adapted from *Jane Brody's Good Food Book* (1985), pp 520–521.

1½ pounds eggplant (2 small), peeled and diced
1 large green pepper, seeded and cut into squares
3 cloves chopped garlic
1½ pounds zucchini, cut into ½ inch slices

¼ cup olive oil
2 large onions, thickly sliced
1 large sweet red pepper, seeded and cut into squares
2½ pounds ripe tomatoes, peeled, seeded and coarsely chopped
1 teaspoon of ground cumin, 1 teaspoon

⅛ teaspoon of cayenne

of turmeric, and ½ teaspoon of coriander

1. Cut the eggplant into ¾-inch cubes.
2. Heat the oil in a large, cast iron skillet. Add onions and green and red peppers and sauté until the onions are translucent. Add chopped garlic and tomatoes. Cook the vegetables, stirring for about 3 minutes. Transfer to a large pot or Dutch oven.
3. Heat another tablespoon of oil and sauté the zucchini for about 10 minutes. Add the zucchini to other vegetables in the pot.
4. Add oil to skillet and sauté the eggplant for about 10 minutes.
5. Mix the vegetables. Heat the ratatouille, cook for about 5 minutes. Stir in herbs and salt to taste.

TURMERIC
(Curcuma longa)

Historical Uses

Turmeric was used internally to regulate blood sugar in diabetics and to prevent colon cancer. It was applied topically as a paste to reduce canker sores and cold sores. It was also used as a yellow dye for the robes of Buddist monks. Turmeric is also known as Indian saffron or yellow ginger.

Growth

A member of the ginger family, turmeric is a perennial plant cultivated in tropical regions of Asia (McCaleb et al., 2000).

Part Used

• Root

Major Chemical Compounds

• Curcumin
• Volatile oils
• Tumerone
• Atlantone and zingiberone sugars
• Resins
• Proteins
• Vitamins and minerals (Leung,1980; Ammon & Wahl, 1991).

Clinical Uses

Turmeric inhibits cancer, has anti-inflammatory and antioxidant effects, and lowers cholesterol levels. It is approved by the German Commission E and the World Health Organization for dyspepsia (Blumenthal et al., 2000). It is also used for acne, dermatitis, infections, dandruff, gastritis, gingivitis, herpes, inflammation, sunburn, and psoriasis (Duke, *http://www.ars-grin.gov/duke/*, 2000). It may have anti-HIV effects (DeClercq, 2000).

Mechanism of Action

This herb enhances cortisol levels, lowers cytokine levels, inhibits leukotriene formation (Duke, *http://www.ars-grin.gov/duke/*, 2000), promotes fibrinolysis, and stabilizes

273

cellular membranes (Scrimal & Dhawan, 1979). Curcumin has been proposed as an HIV-1 integrase inhibitor (DeClercq, 2000).

Dosage

Capsules (*standardized turmeric extract of up to 95 percent curcuminoids*): 450-mg capsule three times daily (McCaleb et al., 2000).

Tea decoction: Steep 1.3 grams of turmeric root in 150 mL of boiled water for 10 to 15 minutes and drink twice daily (Blumenthal et al., 2000).

Side Effects

None are known.

Contraindications

- Turmeric is contraindicated in patients with bile duct obstructions because it may increase the output of bile (Blumenthal et al., 1998).
- It is contraindicated in patients with stomach ulcers or hyperacidity (McGuffin et al., 1997).

Herb-Drug Interactions

None are known.

Pregnancy and Breast-Feeding

Turmeric should be avoided by pregnant women except as a normal part of cooking. It may stimulate uterine contractions and promote menstruation (McGuffin et al., 1997).

SUMMARY OF STUDIES

Nagabhushan & Bhide (1992). This study looked at curcumin as an inhibitor of cancer. Results: Curcumin has anticarcinogenic activity because it inhibits replication of fully developed neoplastic cells.

Scrimal & Dhawan (1979). Some pharmacological actions of curcumin have been examined in rats, mice, and cats. This study looked at curcumin as a nonsteroidal anti-inflammatory drug. Results: This compound has significant anti-inflammatory activity in acute and chronic models of inflammation. Curcumin is as effective as cortisone or pheylbutazone in acute inflammation, but only half as potent in chronic conditions. It has much lower ulcerogenic properties than phenylbutazone and it prevents inflammation-induced increases in SGOT and SGPT levels. It has no analgesic or antipyretic activity.

Prucksunand et al. (2001). In this study of 45 subjects with peptic ulcers, two turmeric capsules of 300 mg each five times a day improved symptoms within the first few weeks of treatment.

REFERENCES

Ammon, H., & Wahl, M (1991). Pharmacology of Curcuma longa. *Planta Medica, 57,*1–7.

Blumenthal, M., Goldberg, A., & Brinckmann, J. (Eds.). (2000). *Herbal medicine expanded Commission E monographs* (pp. 379–384). Austin, TX: American Botanical Council; Newton, MA: Integrative Medicine Communications.

Blumenthal, M., Busse, W., Goldberg, A., Gruenwald, J., Hall, T., Riggins, C., & Rister, R. (Eds.). (1998). *The complete German Commission E monographs: Therapeutic guide to herbal medicines.* (S. Klein & R. Rister, Trans.). Austin, TX: American Botanical Council; Newton, MA: Integrative Medicine Communications.

Carlson, C. (July/August 2000). Turmeric : The gold standard of spices. *Herbs for Health,* 60–64.

DeClercq, E. (2000). Current lead natural products for the chemotherapy of human immunodeficiency virus (HIV) infection. *Medicinal Research Reviews, 20*(5), 323–349.

Duke, J. (2000) Phytochemical and Ethnobotanical Database at the Agricultural Research Services.

Leung, A. (1980). *Encyclopedia of common natural ingredients used in foods, drugs and cosmetics* (pp. 313–314). New York: John Wiley & Sons.

McCaleb, R., Leigh, E., & Morien, K. (2000). *The Encyclopedia of Popular Herbs.* Roseville, CA: Prima Publishing.

McGuffin, M., Hobbs, C., Upton, R., & Goldberg, A. (1997). *Botanical Safety Handbook* (p. 39), Boca Raton, FL: CRC Press.

Nagabhushan, N., & Bhide, S. (1992). Curcumin as an inhibitor of cancer. *Journal of the American College of Nutrition, 11,* 192–198.

Prucksunand, C., Indrasukhsri, B., Leethochawalit, M., & Hungspreugs, K. (2001). Phase II clinical trial on effect of the long turmeric (Curcuma longa Linn) on healing of peptic ulcer. *The Southeast Asian Journal of Tropical Medicine and Public Health, 32*(1), 208–215.

Scrimal, R., & Dhawan, B. (1973). Pharmacology of diferuloyl methane (curcumin), a non-steroidal anti-inflammatory agent. *Journal of Pharmacy and Pharmacology, 25,* 447–452.

NOTES

NOTES

TURMERIC
(Curcuma longa)

Historical Uses

Turmeric was used internally to regulate blood sugar in diabetics and to prevent colon cancer. It was applied topically as a paste to reduce canker sores and cold sores. It was also used as a yellow dye for the robes of Buddist monks. Turmeric is also known as Indian saffron or yellow ginger.

Growth

A member of the ginger family, turmeric is a perennial plant cultivated in tropical regions of Asia.

Part Used

• Root

Medical Uses

Turmeric inhibits cancer, has anti-inflammatory and antioxidant effects, and lowers cholesterol levels. It may be used for stomach upset, acne, dermatitis, infections, dandruff, gastritis, gingivitis, herpes, inflammation, sunburn, and psoriasis.

Dosage

Capsules (standardized turmeric extract of up to 95 percent curcuminoids): 450-mg capsule three times daily.

Tea decoction: Steep 1.3 gram of turmeric root in 150 mL of boiled water for 10 to 15 minutes and drink twice daily.

Warnings

• Don't take turmeric if you have gallbladder problems, stomach ulcers, or other stomach problems. Consult your health-care practitioner.
• Don't use turmeric during pregnancy except as a normal part of cooking. Turmeric in large amounts may stimulate uterine contractions and promote menstruation.

RECIPES

Turmeric is used as a seasoning in cooking and is the highest known source of beta carotene. Store it in the refrigerator and add it at the end of cooking to preserve its medicinal qualities. Use turmeric as a marinade before grilling food to reduce the carcinogens created by grilling. Acids such as vinegar and lemon help to stabilize curcumin.

ANTI-OXIDANT CURRY POWDER

Mix 1 tablespoon of turmeric with ½ teaspoon of cardamom, ¼ teaspoon of cloves, ¼ teaspoon of cumin, ½ teaspoon of coriander, ⅛ teaspoon of celery seed, and ½ teaspoon of cinnamon. Use this curry powder to season rice, chicken, and lentil soup.

CURRIED RICE

Cook 2 cups of basmati rice in 4 cups of water for about 10 minutes while preparing vegetables. In a skillet, sauté two onions, four cloves of garlic, two tablespoons of ginger, five teaspoons of curry powder, and ½ teaspoon of salt in olive oil. Add 1 chopped green pepper and 1 chopped red pepper and continue sautéing. Add the rice mixture and cook until the rice turns yellow from the curry. This is a colorful, festive dish that contains quercetin and flavonoids (onions), vitamins (peppers), and antioxidant effects (curry). It serves 6.

VALERIAN
(Valeriana officinalis)

Historical Uses

The Greeks, Romans, and English colonists used valerian for sleep problems, digestive problems, and menstrual cramps (McCaleb, 2000). It has also been called garden heliotrope.

Growth

Native to Europe and North America, valerian will grow in New England herb gardens. It loves wet soil. Its stems can grow to 5 feet tall, and the petite flowers make up a flower head with small, fragrant pink and white flowers. The roots are harvested in the spring and fall. Unfortunately, they smell like dirty socks.

Part Used

• Root

Major Chemical Compounds

• 0.8 to 1 percent valeric acid
• 1.0 to 1.5 percent valtrate
• Volatile oils

Clinical Uses

Valerian is used for anxiety, stress, insomnia, and hypertension in which anxiety is a factor. It is approved by the German Commission E for "restlessness and sleeping disorders based on nervous conditions." It is approved by the World Health Organization for "sedative and sleep-promoting properties" (Blumenthal et al., 2000). Valerian is generally regarded as safe and is approved for food use by the Food and Drug Administration.

Mechanism of Action

In animal studies, valerian and benzodiazepines bind to gamma-aminobutyric acid-A receptors to cause sedation (Mennini et al., 1993). Valerian's active compounds have a weaker effect than diazepam (Valium) or alprazolam (Xanax). There is no risk of dependence or addiction as there is with benzodiazepines. Valerian decreases the time it takes to get to sleep and reduces nighttime awakenings.

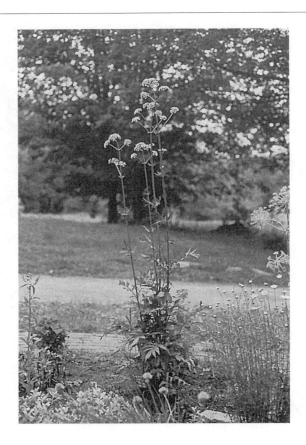

Dosage

Controversy exists over which chemical compound should be used to standard-ize valerian; therefore, it is standardized to 0.8 to 1 percent valerenic acid or 1 to 1.5 percent valtrate or 0.5 percent essential oil (McCaleb et al., 2000). It may take 6 to 8 weeks to see the effects of the herb. Valerian combines well in teas and tinctures with other anti-anxiety herbs such as chamomile and lemon balm.

Standardized extract: 300–400 mg a day (McCaleb et al., 2000). Take 30 minutes to 1 hour before bedtime.

Tea: Pour 1 cup of boiling water over 1 to 2 teaspoons of the root and infuse for 10 to 15 minutes. Keep covered while steeping to preserve the volatile oils. Drink up to 2 cups a day.

Tincture: Start with the lowest dosage of 1 to 3 mL (½ to 1 teaspoon) up to three times daily (Blumenthal et al., 2000).

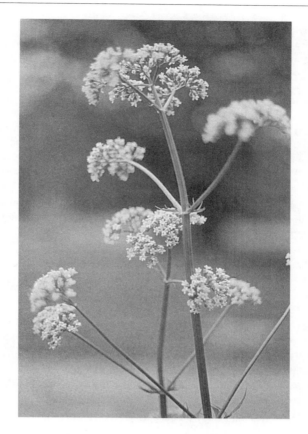

Side Effects

Valerian may cause mild stomach upset. A small number of people who have tried valerian have experienced excitement and irritability rather than relaxation.

Contraindications

- A standardized extract should always be used.
- Patients should not drive or operate machinery after consuming valerian (McGuffin et al., 1997).
- Some research indicates that continuous high doses may lead to headaches and palpitations. Patients who develop these symptoms should take frequent breaks from valerian (every 2 to 3 weeks).

Herb-Drug Interactions

Valerian may potentiate barbiturates (Upton, 1999) and increase sedation (Miller, 1998). Advise patients against consuming alcohol while taking valerian (McCaleb et al., 2000).

Pregnancy and Breast-Feeding

Valerian is safe at the recommended dosage (McGuffin et al., 1997).

 # SUMMARY OF STUDIES

Cerny et al. (1999). This double-blind, placebo-controlled, multicenter study included 88 healthy volunteers who did not have insomnia. They took a valerian-lemon balm combination (Songha Night from Switzerland containing 480 mg valerian dry extract [4.5:1] and 240 mg lemon balm dry extract [5:1]) 30 minutes before bed. Results: Subjects who took the valerian combination had a much greater improvement in sleep quality without serious side effects.

Willey et al. (1995). In this valerian overdose case report, an 18-year-old woman ingested 40 to 50 470-mg capsules of 100 percent powdered valerian root in a suicide attempt. She presented with mild symptoms, all of which resolved within 24 hours. Valerian overdose, at about 20 times the recommended therapeutic dose, appears to be benign.

Lindahl & Lindwall (1988). This double-blind study included 27 subjects. Results: Compared with placebo, valerian showed a good and significant effect on poor sleep; 44 percent of patients reported perfect sleep, and 89 percent reported improved sleep. No side effects were reported.

Balderer & Borbely (1985). This double-blind, crossover study included 18 subjects. Results: Aqueous valerian extract exerts a mild hypnotic action and significant sleep-promoting action.

Leathwood et al. (1981). This study included 128 subjects. Results: Valerian produced a significant decrease in subjectively evaluated sleep latency scores and significant improvement in sleep quality. Women and younger people who define themselves as habitually poor or irregular sleepers were most sensitive to valerian.

Fussel et al. (2000). In this pilot study, 30 patients suffering from mild to moderate insomnia were given a combination extract of valerian 250 mg and hop extract 60 mg and reported improvements in sleep after 2 weeks.

Donath et al. (2000). In this randomized, double-blind, placebo-controlled crossover study, 16 subjects with mild insomnia took valerian extract for 14 days and reported an improvement in sleep with a low number of adverse effects.

REFERENCES

Balderer, G., & Borbely, A. (1985). Effect of valerian on human sleep. *Psychopharmacology, 87,* 406–409.

Blumenthal, M., Goldberg, A., & Brinckmann, J. (Eds.). (2000). *Herbal medicine expanded Commission E monographs* (pp. 394–399, 487). Austin, TX: American Botanical Council; Newton, MA: Integrative Medicine Communications.

A. (1985). Effect of valerian on human sleep. *Psychopharmacology,* 87:406–409.

Cerny, A., & Schmid, K. (1999). Tolerability and efficacy of valerian/lemon balm in healthy volunteers (a double-blind, placebo-controlled, multicentre study). *Filoterapia, 70,* 221–228.

Donath, F., Quispe, S., Diefenbach, K., Maurer, A., Fietze, I., and Roots, I. (2000). Critical evaluation of the effect of valerian extract on sleep structure and sleep quality. *Pharmacopsychiatry, 33*(2), 47–53.

Fussel, A., Wolf, A., & Brattstrom, A. (2000). Effect of a fixed valerian-hop extract combination (Ze91019) on sleep polygraphy in patients with non-organic insomnia: A pilot study. *European Journal of Medical Research, 5*(9), 385–390.

Leathwood, P., Chafford, F., Heck, E., & Munoz-Box, R. (1982). Aqueous extract of valerian root (*Valeriana officinalis L.*) improves sleep quality in man. *Pharmacology, Biochemistry and Behavior, 17*, 65–71.

Lindahl, O., & Lindwall, L. (1989). Double blind study of a valerian preparation. *Pharmacology, Biochemistry and Behavior, 32*(4),1065–1066.

McCaleb, R., Leigh, E., & Morien, K. (2000). *The Encyclopedia of Popular Herbs.* Roseville, CA: Prima Publishing.

McGuffin, M., Hobbs, C., Upton, R., & Goldberg, A. (1997). *Botanical Safety Handbook* (p. 120). Boca Raton, FL: CRC Press.

Mennini, T., et al. (1993). In vitro study on the interaction of extracts and pure compounds from *Valeriana officinalis* roots with GABA, benzodiazepine and barbiturate receptors in rat brain. *Filoterapia, 54*, 291–300.

Miller, L. (1998). Herbal medicinals: Selected clinical considerations focusing on known or potential drug-herb interactions. *Archives of Internal Medicine, 158*, 2200–2211. Cited in Vickers & Zollman (1999). Herbal medicine. *British Medical Journal, 319*, 1050–1053.

Ody, P. (1993). *The complete medicinal herbal.* New York: Dorling Kindersley Publishing.

Upton, R. (Ed.) (1999). Valerian (*Valerian officinalis*). *American herbal* CA: Soquel.

Willey, L., Mady, S., Cobaugh, D., & Wax, P. (1995). Valerian overdose: A case report. *Veterinarian and Human Toxicology, 37*(4), 364–365.

NOTES

NOTES

VALERIAN
(Valeriana officinalis)

Historical Uses

The Greeks, Romans, and English colonists used valerian for sleep problems, digestive problems, and menstrual cramps. It has also been called garden heliotrope.

Growth

Native to Europe and North America, valerian will grow in New England herb gardens. It loves wet soil. Its stems can grow to 5 feet tall, and the petite flowers make up a flower head with small, fragrant pink and white flowers. The roots are harvested in the spring and fall. Unfortunately, they smell like dirty socks.

Part Used

• Root

Medical Uses

Valerian is used for anxiety, stress, insomnia, and hypertension in which anxiety is a factor.

Dosage

Controversy exists over which chemical compound should be used to standardize valerian; therefore, it is standardized to 0.8 to 1 percent valerenic acid or 1 to 1.5 percent valtrate or 0.5 percent essential oil. It may take 6 to 8 weeks to see the effects of the herb. Valerian combines well in teas and tinctures with other antianxiety herbs such as chamomile and lemon balm.

Standardized extract: 300–400 mg a day. Take 30 minutes to 1 hour before bedtime.

Tea: Pour 1 cup of boiling water over 1 to 2 teaspoon of the root and infuse for 10 to 15 minutes. Keep covered while steeping to preserve the volatile oils. Drink up to 2 cups a day.

Tincture: Start with the lowest dosage of 1 to 3 mL ($\frac{1}{2}$ to 1 teaspoon) up to three times daily.

Warnings

• Valerian may cause mild stomach upset.

- Asmall number of people who have tried valerian have experienced excitement and irritability rather than relaxation.
- Some research indicates that continuous high doses of valerian may lead to headaches and an irregular heartbeat. Report any side effects to your health-care practitioner.
- Valerian is generally regarded as safe and is approved for food use by the Food and Drug Administration. Always use standardized extract.
- Don't drive or operate machinery after taking valerian.
- Don't take valerian with barbiturates or when drinking alcohol.
- Valerian is safe during pregnancy and breast-feeding at the recommended dosage.

STRESS REDUCERS

If you have an anxiety-related condition, try these stress-reduction "recipes" to help yourself relax, increase the oxygen flow in your body, and decrease your heart rate.

Belly Breathing. While lying or sitting, close your eyes and place both hands on your belly. As you breathe in through your nose, feel your stomach push out into your hands. As you breathe out through your mouth, feel your stomach pull in. Try this three times. Then hold your breath for a few seconds and enjoy this peaceful, restful time.

If you have trouble going to sleep at night, do a few belly breaths with your eyes closed. If thoughts come into your mind, just start counting each breath as you exhale. If you still have trouble going to sleep, play an audiotape of the sounds of gentle waves. Inhale as each wave recedes, and exhale as each wave comes to shore.

Exercise. Get some form of exercise daily, such as a meditative walk. Or try lying face up with your back on a huge exercise ball; relax to help stretch your stomach area. During your exercise time, be sure to get plenty of sunshine and fresh air.

Meditation. Either lie down or sit comfortably in a chair with your feet flat on the floor and your hands in your lap. Make sure the room is quiet, the phone is off the hook, and the door is closed. Or go for a quiet walk in the woods and lean up against a tree. Close your eyes. Take a deep breath in through your nose and breathe out through your mouth. As you inhale, feel your stomach push out. As you exhale, feel your stomach pull in. Relax, and think of a peaceful image. Or, if you choose, think of a word such as "peace" or "love" and repeat that in your mind. Relax for about 10 minutes. Do this exercise at least once a day.

WITCH HAZEL
(Hamamelis virginiana)

Historical Uses

In folklore, witch hazel was used externally for inflammation and hemorrhoids. It is still available over the counter in pharmacies and is present in most home medicine chests.

Growth

Witch hazel is an ornamental tree with yellow flowers that have narrow petals. It grows wild in forests from Canada to Florida.

Parts Used

- Leaves
- Bark

Major Chemical Compounds

- Tannins (found more in leaves than in bark)
- Gallic acid
- Bitters

Clinical Uses

Witch hazel may be used for hemorrhoids, varicose veins, sprains, bruises, muscle aches, scrapes, and sunburn. It is approved by the German Commission E for "minor skin injuries, local inflammation of the skin and mucous membranes, hemorrhoids and varicose veins" (Blumenthal et al., 2000).

Mechanism of Action

Astringent properties result from tannins in the leaves and bark (Tyler, 1993). They control bleeding and reduce inflammation (Foster & Duke, 1990).

Dosage

Undistilled or unrefined witch hazel: Use this form of witch hazel externally three to four times daily. It also may be used as a gel, an ointment, a lotion, or a salve.

Decoction of bark: For external use, place 2 to 3 grams of powdered bark in 150 mL cold water and boil for 10 to 15 minutes, cool (Blumenthal, et al., 2000).

287

Compress: Dip a clean cloth or gauze into the warm decoction and apply to affected area three or four times daily.

Poultice: Place the warm herb in clean gauze and apply externally to the inflamed area.

Side Effects

Some patients who take witch hazel internally develop irritation of the stomach. Witch hazel tannins may cause liver damage (McGuffin et al., 1997).

Contraindications

• None are known.

Herb-Drug Interactions

None are known.

Pregnancy and Breast-Feeding

External use of witch hazel is safe during pregnancy and breast-feeding (McGuffin et al., 1997).

 # SUMMARY OF STUDIES

Recent clinical studies in humans are limited.

REFERENCES

Blumenthal, M., Goldberg, A., & Brinckmann, J. (Eds.). (2000). *Herbal medicine expanded Commission E monographs* (pp 413–418). Austin, TX: American Botanical Council; Newton, MA: Integrative Medicine Communications.

Foster, S., & Duke, J. (1990). *Eastern/central medicinal plants* (p. 256). New York: Houghton Mifflin.

Hoffman, D. (1994). *The information sourcebook of herbal medicine* (p. 160). Freedom, CA: The Crossing Press.

McGuffin, M., Hobbs, C., Upton, R., & Goldberg, A. (1997). *Botanical Safety Handbook* (pp. 59–60, 120). Boca Raton, FL: CRC Press.

Tyler, V. (1993). *The honest herbal* (pp. 319–320. Binghamton, NY: Pharmaceutical Products Press.

NOTES

WITCH HAZEL
(Hamamelis virginiana)

Historical Uses

In folklore, witch hazel was used externally for inflammation and hemorrhoids. It is still available over the counter in pharmacies and is present in most home medicine chests.

Growth

Witch hazel is an ornamental tree with yellow flowers that have narrow petals. It grows wild in forests from Canada to Florida.

Parts Used

- Leaves
- Bark

Medical Uses

Witch hazel may be used for hemorrhoids, varicose veins, sprains, bruises, muscle aches, scrapes, and sunburn.

Dosage

Undistilled or unrefined witch hazel: Use this form of witch hazel externally three to four times daily. It may also be used as a gel, an ointment, a lotion, or a salve.

Decoction of bark: For external use, place 2 to 3 grams of powdered bark in 150 mL cold water and boil for 10 to 15 minutes, cool.

Compress: Dip a clean cloth or gauze into the warm decoction and apply to the affected area three or four times daily.

Poultice: Place the warm herb in clean gauze and apply externally to the inflamed area.

Warnings

- Some people who take witch hazel internally develop irritation of the stomach.
- Witch hazel tannins may cause liver damage.
- External use of witch hazel is safe during pregnancy and breast-feeding.

RECIPES

WITCH HAZEL OINTMENT

Simmer 2 tablespoons of witch hazel leaves in about 7 ounces of petroleum or nonpetroleum jelly for about 10 minutes. Strain the herb out and place the ointment in jars. Label and date the jars.

CLEANSING WITCH HAZEL LOTION

Mix 1½ tablespoons of witch hazel with 1 tablespoon of glycerine, apply it to your face, and then rinse.

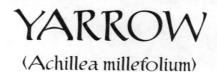

YARROW
(Achillea millefolium)

Historical Uses

Yarrow was called "soldiers' woundwort" because the leaves were taken onto the battlefield and applied to stop wounds from bleeding. Yarrow compresses were used for hemorrhoids. In folklore, fresh yarrow root was used as an anesthetic for surgery (Weiss, 1985). Fresh roots or leaves were also mashed in whiskey and used for toothache (Weiss, 1985).

Growth

Yarrow grows wild in meadows and on roadsides in North America. The flower heads grow in clusters of different-colored varieties of white, yellow, orange, and bright red. White yarrow is the variety most often used medicinally (Weiss, 1985). Yarrow repels ants, flies, Japanese beetles, and termites (Weiss, 1985).

Part Used

• Flowers (whole white flower heads)

Major Chemical Compounds

• Tannins
• Volatile oils
• Flavonoids
• Vitamins (ascorbic acid, folic acid)
• Coumarins

Clinical Uses

Yarrow encourages perspiration, appetite, and strength. It is approved by the German Commission E for loss of appetite and dyspepsia and externally for psychosomatic cramps of the female pelvis (Blumenthal et al., 2000).

Mechanism of Action

The anti-inflammatory and antispasmodic properties of yarrow may result from its flavonoid content (Bruneton, 1995).

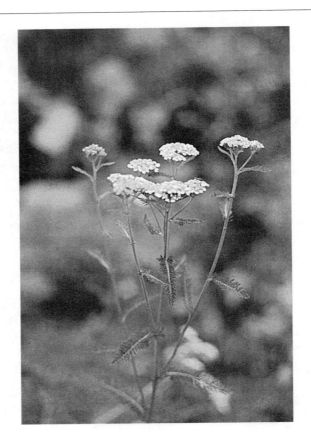

Dosage

Tincture 1:5: 1 teaspoon three times a day between meals (Blumenthal et al., 2000).

Tea by infusion: Pour 1 cup of boiling water onto 1 to 2 teaspoons of dried yarrow and infuse for 10 to 15 minutes. Drink three times a day between meals (Hoffman, 1992).

Bath: Place flower heads in the bath water to reduce a fever.

Sitz bath: Use 100 grams of yarrow per 5 gallons of warm water. Have patient sit in bath for 10 to 20 minutes and then rinse (Blumenthal et al., 2000).

Side Effects

None are known.

Contraindications

- Yarrow is contraindicated in people with allergies to Asteraceae (McGuffin et al., 1997).

- Federal regulations state that foods or beverages containing yarrow must be thujone-free (McGuffin et al., 1997).

Pregnancy and Breast-Feeding

Yarrow should not be taken internally during pregnancy because it may stimulate the uterus and menstruation (McGuffin et al., 1997). No restrictions are known for breast-feeding (Blumenthal et al., 2000).

Herb-Drug Interactions

None are known.

 # SUMMARY OF STUDIES

No recent clinical studies in humans are available.

REFERENCES

Blumenthal, M., Goldberg, A., & Brinckmann, J. (Eds.). (2000). *Herbal medicine expanded Commission E monographs* (pp. 419–423). Austin, TX: American Botanical Council; Newton, MA: Integrative Medicine Communications.

Bruneton, J. (1995). *Pharmacognosy, Phytochemistry, Medicinal Plants.* Paris: Lavoisier Publishing. Cited in: M. Blumenthal, A. Goldberg, & J. Brinckmann (Eds.). (2000). *Herbal Medicine Expanded Commission E Monographs* (pp. 379–384). Austin, Tex: American Botanical Council; Boston: Integrative Medicine Communications.

Hoffman, D. (1992). *The new holistic herbal.* Boston: Element Books Limited.

McGuffin, M., Hobbs, C., Upton, R., & Goldberg, A. (1997). *Botanical Safety Handbook* (p. 6). Boca Raton, FL: CRC Press.

Weiss, G., & Weiss, S. (1985). *Growing and using the healing herbs* (pp. 235–236). Emmaus, PA: Rodale Press.

NOTES

NOTES

YARROW
(Achillea millefolium)

Historical Uses

Yarrow was called "soldiers' woundwort" because the leaves were taken onto the battlefied and applied to stop wounds from bleeding. Yarrow compresses were used for hemorrhoids. In folklore, fresh yarrow root was used as an anesthetic for surgery. Fresh roots or leaves were also mashed in whiskey and used for toothache.

Growth

Yarrow grows wild in meadows and on roadsides in North America. The flower heads grow in clusters of different-colored varieties of white, yellow, orange, and bright red. White yarrow is the variety most often used medicinally. Yarrow repels ants, flies, Japanese beetles, and termites.

Part Used

- Flowers (whole white flower heads)

Medical Uses

Yarrow encourages perspiration, appetite, and strength.

Dosage

Tincture 1:5: 1 teaspoon three times a day between meals (Blumenthal et al., 2000).

Tea by infusion: Pour 1 cup of boiling water onto 1 to 2 teaspoons of dried yarrow and infuse for 10 to 15 minutes. Drink three times a day between meals (Hoffman, 1992).

Bath: Place flower heads in the bath water to reduce a fever.

Sitz bath: Use 100 grams of yarrow per 5 gallons of warm water. Have patient sit in bath for 10 to 20 minutes and then rinse (Blumenthal et al., 2000).

Warnings

- Don't use yarrow if you are allergic to Asteraceae.
- Don't take yarrow internally if you are pregnant because it may stimulate the uterus and menstruation.

APPENDICES, REFERENCES, AND RESOURCES

Appendix 1

QUICK GUIDE TO HERB-DRUG INTERACTIONS

The rapid increase in the use of herbal medicines has created a rapidly growing database of known herb-drug interactions, many of which are presented in the table below. Keep in mind, however, that our knowledge of the interactions among prescription medicines, over-the-counter medicines, and herbal medicines continues to change constantly.

To help detect possible herb-drug interactions, encourage patients to be open about all medicines they may be taking, whether prescription, over the counter, or herbal. Ask them to bring all of their medications with them to their next appointment. Caution patients not to take herbal medicines in higher doses or more often than recommended. Also, caution them not to experiment with herbal medicines. Urge them to tell all of their health-care practitioners about all of the medicines they take.

If patients are known to have adverse drug reactions, such as allergies, chronic skin rashes, or pre-existing liver disease related to prescription medicines, warn them that they have a higher risk of side effects from herbs as well. Reinforce the importance of reporting any side effects of prescription, over-the-counter, and herbal medicines to a health-care practitioner. Elderly patients, pregnant women, and children have an increased risk of interactions and side effects from herbal medicines and should be referred to a practitioner with specialized training in the field of herbal medicine. Also, make a point of telling pregnant women that some herbs are unsafe to take during pregnancy and breast-feeding.

HERB	DRUG	INTERACTION	SOURCE OF INFORMATION
ALOE GEL/JUICE	Glyburide	Increased hypo-glycemic effect	Yongchaiyudha et al., 1996
ALOE LATEX	Antiarrhythmics Cardiac glycosides Corticosteroids Licorice root Thiazide diuretics	May potentiate the action of cardiac glyco-sides and anti-arrhythmic agents (as do the other drugs listed)	Blumenthal et al., 1998
ASTRAGALUS ROOT	Acyclovir Interleukin-2	Increases effects	DeSmet & D'Arcy, 1996
	Azathioprine Cyclosporine Methotrexate	Caution use	
BITTER MELON	Chlorpropamide	Increases hypo-glycemic effect	Aslam & Stockley, 1979
BORAGE	Anticonvulsants	May lower seizure threshold	Miller, 1998
BROMELAIN	Anticoagulants	Increases bleeding	Blumenthal et al., 1998
	Tetracycline	Increases plasma and urine drug levels	Neurauer, 1961
	Chloramphenicol Erythromycin Novobiocin Penicillin	Enhances drug levels	Neurauer, 1961
	5-fluorouracil Vincristine	Can improve efficacy	Taussig & Batkin, 1998
BREWER'S YEAST	MAO inhibitors	Increased blood pressure	Blumenthal et al., 1998
BUCKTHORN BARK, BERRY	Cardiac glyco-sides Quinidine	May potentiate toxicity with long-term use	Blumenthal et al., 2000
BUGLEWEED	Thyroid preparations Thyroid treatments	Contraindicated	Blumenthal et al., 1998 McGuffin et al., 1997

HERB	DRUG	INTERACTION	SOURCE OF INFORMATION
BUPLEURUM	Alcohol CNS depressants Sedatives	May increase sedation	WHO, 1999
CASCARA SAGRADA BARK	Cardiac glyco- sides Quinidine	May potentiate toxicity with long-term use	Blumenthal et al., 2000
CHASTE TREE BERRY	Dopamine- receptor antag- onists (such as haloperidol)	May weaken effect (animal studies)	Blumenthal et al., 1998
	Metoclopramide	Possible inter- actions	Blumenthal et al., 2000
	Hormone therapy Oral contracep- tives	Contraindicated	Blumenthal et al., 2000
CAYENNE PEPPER	Aspirin	Reduced mucosal damage if cayenne taken 30 minutes before aspirin	Yeoh et al., 1995
CINCHONA BARK	Anticoagulants	Increases effects	Blumenthal et al., 1998
COLA NUT	Caffeine Psychoanaleptic drugs	Contraindicated	Blumenthal et al., 1998
DEVIL'S CLAW ROOT	Antiarrhythmics	Contraindicated	ESCOP, 1999
DONG QUAI	Coumadin	May increase effects of medication	Heck et al., 2000
ECHINACEA	Amiodarone Anabolic steroids Ketoconazole Methotrexate	If >8 weeks, potential for hepatotoxicity	Miller, 1998
	Corticosteroids Cyclosporin	Antagonistic effects	
EPHEDRA (MA HUANG)	Cardiac glyco- sides Halothane	Cardiac arrhyth- mias	Blumenthal et al., 1998
	Guanethidine	Enhances sympa- thomimetic effect	Blumenthal et al., 1998

HERB	DRUG	INTERACTION	SOURCE OF INFORMATION
	MAO inhibitors	May cause fatal hypertension	Blumenthal et al., 1998
	Ergotamine Oxytocin	Hypertension	WHO, 1999
EUCALYPTUS OIL (EXTERNAL OR INHALED)	Drugs weakened or shortened	Affects liver detoxification	Blumenthal et al., 2000
EVENING PRIMROSE OIL	Anticonvulsants	May lower seizure threshold	Miller, 1998
FENNEL	Ciprofloxacin	Affects absorption, distribution, elimination	Zhu et al., 1999
FENUGREEK	Hypoglycemic agents Sulfonylureas	May exaggerate effects	*Natural Medicines,* 2000
FEVERFEW	Aspirin Coumadin	May increase bleeding time	Herbst, 1999 Miller, 1998
	Nonsteroidal anti-inflammatory drugs	Inhibits effects of herb	Miller, 1998
FLAXSEED	Conventional medicines	May delay absorption	Blumenthal et al., 1998
	Antidiabetic medications	May slow glucose absorption	Blumenthal, 2000
GARLIC	Coumadin	May increase bleeding time	Sunter, 1991 Herbst, 1999 Miller, 1998 Ottariano, 1999
GINGER	Anticoagulants	May increase bleeding time	Lumb, 1994 Herbst, 1999 Miller, 1998
GINKGO BILOBA	Aspirin Coumadin	May increase bleeding time	Rosenblatt, 1997 Herbst, 1999 Miller, 1998
	Papaverine	May potentiate effects of drug	Sikora et al., 1989
	Trazodone	May cause severe CNS depression	*Prescriber's Letter,* September 2000

301

HERB	DRUG	INTERACTION	SOURCE OF INFORMATION
GREEN TEA	Coumadin	May increase effects	Heck et al., 2000
GURMAR LEAVES	Glyburide Tolbutamide	May have additive effects	Baskaran et al., 1990
	Insulin	May reduce insulin requirements	Shanmugasundaram et al., 1990
HAWTHORN LEAF WITH FLOWER	Cardiac glycosides	May enhance effects of drug	Blumenthal, 2000
	Adenosine Caffeine Epinephrine Papaverine Sodium nitrate Theophylline	May increase coronary artery dilatation (controversial)	Blumenthal, 2000
	Digoxin	May affect drug level monitoring	Miller, 1998
KARELA	Biguanides Insulin Sulphonylureas	May cause interactions	Miller, 1998
KAVA KAVA	Alcohol Barbiturates Benzodiazepines	May potentiate effects	Herbst, 1999
	Levodopa	May reduce effects	Schelosky et al., 1995
LICORICE ROOT	Spironolactone	May increase loss of potassium	WHO, 1999 Miller, 1998
	Amiloride Cardiac glycosides Thiazide diuretics	May increase loss of potassium	WHO, 1999
	Digoxin	May create problems with drug monitoring	Miller, 1998
MARSHMALLOW LEAF AND ROOT	All	May decrease absorption of medications	Blumenthal et al., 1998
OAK BARK	All	May decrease absorption of medications	Blumenthal et al., 1998

HERB	DRUG	INTERACTION	SOURCE OF INFORMATION
PAPAYA	Coumadin	Increases effect of medication	Shulman, 1997
PANAX GINSENG	MAO inhibitors Phenelzine	May interact	Blumenthal et al., 1998 Miller, 1998
	Coumadin	May alter bleeding times	Miller, 1998
	Corticosteroids Estrogens	May have additive effects	Miller, 1998
	Digoxin	May affect drug levels	Miller, 1998
	Biguanides Insulin Sulfonylureas	Should not administer together	Miller, 1998
PSYLLIUM	Conventional medicines	May delay absorption	Blumenthal et al., 1998
	Antidiabetic drugs	May slow glucose absorption	Blumenthal et al., 1998
RHUBARB ROOT	Antiarrhythmics Cardiac glyco-sides Corticoadrenal steroids Thiazide diuretics	Increases toxic effects	WHO, 1999
SARSAPARILLA ROOT	Bismuth Digitalis glyco-sides	Increases absorption	Blumenthal et al., 1998
	Hypnotics	Accelerates elimination	Blumenthal et al., 1998
SAW PALMETTO	Iron	May limit absorption	Miller, 1998
SCOTCH BROOM	MAO inhibitors	May cause hyper-tensive crisis	Blumenthal, 2000
SENNA	Cardiac glyco-sides Quinidine	Long-term use can increase loss of serum potassium	Blumenthal, 2000
SIBERIAN GINSENG	Kanamycin Monomycin	May enhance effects of drugs	Vereshchagin et al., 1998
STINGING NETTLES	Diclofenac	Increased anti-inflammatory effects	Chrubasik et al., 1997

HERB	DRUG	INTERACTION	SOURCE OF INFORMATION
ST. JOHN'S WORT	Selective serotonin reuptake inhibitors	Nausea, headache, tremors	Lantz et al., 1999 Roundtree, 2001
	Anticonvulsants Antifungals Antiretrovirals Calcium channel blockers Chemotherapeutics Cyclosporine Macrolide antibiotics Nonsedating antihistamines Oral contraceptives Warfarin	Contraindicated because of possible breakthrough bleeding, lowered blood levels, decreased drug effectiveness	Roby et al., 2000 Piscitelli et al., 2000
	Tetracycline	Increased risk of blood clots	Herbst, 1999
	Iron	May limit absorption	Miller, 1998
VALERIAN	Alcohol Barbiturates	May potentiate effects	Upton, 1999 Herbst, 1999 McCaleb et al., 2000

*The Food and Drug Administration has a list of unsafe herbs. The Internet address is:
http://lep.cl.msu.edu/msueimp/htdoc/modO3/03900066.html

Appendix 2

HERBS THAT MAY INCREASE CLOTTING TIMES OR INTERACT WITH ANTICOAGULANTS

- Astragalus
- Bilberry
- Bromelain
- Capsaicin
- Dong quai
- Evening primrose oil
- Feverfew
- Garlic
- Ginger

- Ginkgo biloba
- Ginseng
- Green tea
- Horse chestnut
- Red clover
- Skullcap
- Sheep sorrel
- Willow bark

Sources: Heck et al., 2000 and Ottariano, 1999.

Appendix 3

HERBS THAT MAY HAVE A LAXATIVE EFFECT

- Aloe latex
- Boneset
- Buckthorn
- Cascara sagrada
- Dandelion root and leaf

- Elder
- Fennel
- Milk thistle
- Psyllium
- Senna

Sources: Ottariano, 1999 and McGuffin, 2000.

Appendix 4

HERBS THAT SHOULD NOT BE TAKEN INTERNALLY

LIVER TOXICITY:
- Comfrey
- Chaparral
- Germander
- Life root

CANCER-CAUSING EFFECTS:
- Sassafras

LIFE-THREATENING TOXICITY IN ANIMALS:
- Pennyroyal oil (has killed some animals after use as a flea repellent.)

Warning: Many plants are toxic and should never be used internally; consult a book on poisonous plants.

Appendix 5

HERBS THAT SHOULD NOT BE TAKEN DURING PREGNANCY

- Agave
- Alder
- Aloe (oral use)
- Angelica
- Buckthorn
- Barberry
- Basil
- Bilberry leaves
- Birthroot
- Blue cohosh root
- Black cohosh
- Black walnut
- Buchu
- Cascara
- Castor oil
- Chaste tree berry
- Coltsfoot
- Comfrey

- Cotton root bark
- Damiana
- Devil's claw root
- Dong quai
- Ephedra
- Ergot
- False unicorn
- Feverfew
- Ginger
- Ginkgo biloba (Egb)
- Ginseng
- Goldenseal
- Gotu kola
- Green tea (caffeine content)
- Hawthorn
- Hops
- Horehound
- Horse chestnut
- Horseradish
- Horsetail
- Hyssop
- Juniper berries
- Kava kava
- Licorice
- Lobelia
- Milk thistle
- Mistletoe
- Mugwort
- Myrrh
- Oregon grape
- Osha
- Pennyroyal leaf, flower, and oil
- Pleurisy root
- Red clover
- Rue leaf
- Rhubarb
- Sarsaparilla
- Scotch broom
- Senna
- Shepherd's purse
- Southernwood
- St. John's wort
- Tansy leaf
- Uva ursi
- Wormwood
- Yarrow
- Yellow dock

Warning: Urge patients to use all herbs cautiously during pregnancy. Some herbs in the list above may induce abortion or stimulate the uterus to contract. Other herbs may have a laxative effect. Advise patients against exceeding recommended dosages, and tell patients to consult with their health-care practitioners about the length of time to take any herbal medicine. For more information on herbs that may or may not be used safely in pregnancy, consult the *Botanical Safety Handbook.*

Appendix 6

HERBS THAT SHOULD NOT BE TAKEN WHILE BREAST-FEEDING

- Aloe (oral use)
- Barberry
- Bilberry leaves
- Black cohosh
- Bladderwrack
- Borage
- Buckthorn
- Bugleweed
- Cascara sagrada
- Chaste tree berry
- Coltsfoot
- Comfrey
- Elecampane
- Ephedra
- Feverfew

- Garlic
- Ginseng
- Goldenseal
- Green tea (caffeine content)
- Hawthorn
- Horse chestnut
- Horseradish
- Hyssop
- Kava kava
- Licorice root
- Psyllium
- Senna
- Stillingia
- Wormwood
- Yellow dock

Warning: Other herbs may be unsafe also. Tell patients to consult a health-care practitioner before taking any herb while breast-feeding.

REFERENCES

Akerele, O. (1992). Summary of WHO guidelines for the assessment of herbal medicines. *Filoterapie*, vol. LXIII, No. 2. Reprinted in *HerbalGram* (*1993*), *28*, 13–16.

Aksel, G., Brask, T., Kambskard, J., & Hentzer, E. (1988). Ginger root against seasickness. *Acta Otolaryngology, 105*, 45–49.

Alternative Medicine Review (2000). Berberine. *5*(2), 175–177.

Amer, M., Taha, M., & Tosson, Z. (1980). The effect of aqueous garlic extract on the growth of dermatophytes. *International Journal of Dermatology, 19*(5), 285–287.

Anderson, J., Johnstone, B., & Cook-Newall, M. (1995). Meta-analysis of the effects of soy protein intake on serum lipids. *New England Journal of Medicine, 333*, 276–282.

Archives of Environmental Health (1987), *42*, 133–136.

Anderson, R. F., Fisher, L. J., Hara, Y., Harris, T., Mak, W. B., Medlton, L. D., & Packer, J. E. (2001). Green tea catechins partially protect DNA from (.)OH radical-induced strand breaks and base damage through fast chemical repair of DNA radicals. *Carcinogenesis, 22*(8), 1189–1193.

Arjmandi, B., Birnbaum, R., Goyal, N., et al. (1998). Bone-sparing effect of soy protein in ovarian hormone-deficient rats is related to its isoflavone content. *American Journal of Clinical Nutrition, 68*(6 Suppl), 1364S–1368S.

Arjmandi, B., Getlinger, M., Goyal, N., Alekel, L., Hasler, C. M., Juma, S., Drum, M. L., Hollis, B. U., & Kukreja, S. C. (1998). Role of soy protein with normal or reduced isoflavone content in reversing bone loss induced by ovarian deficiency in rats. *American Journal of Clinical Nutrition, 68*, 1358S–1363S.

Armanini, D., Bonanni, G., & Palermom (1999). Reduction of serum testosterone in men by licorice. *New England Journal of Medicine, 341*(15), 1158.

Aslam, M., & Stockley, I. (1979). Interaction between curry ingredient (karela) and drug (chlorpropamide) [letter]. *The Lancet, 1*, 607.

Avorn, J, et al. (1994). Reduction of bacteriuria and pyuria after ingestion of cranberry juice. *Journal of the American Medical Association, 271*(10), 751–754.

Awang, D. (1989). Herbal medicine feverfew. *CPJ-RPC*, 266–270.

Backon, J. (1986). Ginger. Inhibition of thromboxane synthetase and stimulation of prostacyclin: Relevance for medicine and psychiatry. *Medical Hypotheses, 20*, 271–278.

Baetgen, D. (1988). Treatment of acute bronchitis in children using Echinacin. *Pediatrie, 1*, 66.

Balderer, G., & Borbely, A. (1985). Effect of valerian on human sleep. *Psychopharmacology, 87*, 406–409.

Bannerjee, B., & Bagchi, D. (2001). Beneficial effects of a novel ih636 grape seed proanthocyanidin extract in the treatment of chronic pancreatitis. *Digestion, 63*(3), 203–206.

Bannermann, J. (1997). Goldenseal in world trade: Pressures and potentials. *HerbalGram, 41*, 51–52.

Baskaran, K, et al. (1990). Use of *Gymnema sylvestre* leaf extract in the control of blood glucose in insulin-dependent diabetes mellitus. *Journal of Ethnopharmacology, 30*, 295–305.

Bassett, I., Pannowitz, D., & Barnetson, R. (1990). A comparative study of tea-tree oil versus benzoylperoxide in the treatment of acne. *Medical Journal of Australia, 153*, 455–458.

Belch, J. J., & Hill, A. (2000). Evening primrose oil and borage oil in rheumatologic conditions. *American Journal of Clinical Nutrition, 71*(1 Suppl), 352S–356S.

Bloomfield, H., Nordfors, M., & McWilliams, P. (1996). *Hypericum and depression.* CA: Prelude. Website at www.hypericum.com

Blumenthal, M. (2000). Interactions between herbs and conventional drugs: Introductory considerations. *HerbalGram, 49*, 52–63.

Blumenthal, M. (1999). Herb market levels after five years of boom: 1999 sales in mainstream market up only 11% in first half of 1999 after 55% increase in 1998. *HerbalGram, 47*, 64–65.

Blumenthal, M. (1997). Industry alert: Plantain adulterated with digitalis. *HerbalGram, 40*, 28–29.

Blumenthal, M., Busse, W., Goldberg, A., Gruenwald, J., Hall, T., Riggins, C., & Rister, R. (Eds.). (1998). *The complete German Commission E monographs: Therapeutic guide to herbal medicines.* (S. Klein & R. Rister, Trans.); Austin, TX: American Botanical Council; Newton, MA: Integrative Medicine Communications.

Blumenthal, M., Goldberg, A., & Brinckmann, J. (Eds.). (2000). *Herbal medicine expanded Commission E monographs;* Austin, TX: American Botanical Council; Newton, MA: Integrative Medicine Communications.

Bone, M., Wilkinson, D., Young, J., & McNeil, J. (1990). Ginger root—A new antiemetic. The effect of ginger root on postoperative nausea and vomiting after major gynaecological surgery. *Anaesthesia, 45*, 669–671.

Bordia, A. (1981). Effect of garlic on blood lipids in patients with coronary heart disease. *American Journal of Clinical Nutrition, 34*, 100–2103.

Bordia, A., Verma, S. K., & Srivastava, K. C. (1997). Effect of ginger (*Zingiber officinale Rosc.*) and fenugreek (*Trigonella foenumgraecum L.*) on blood lipids, blood sugar and platelet aggregation in patients with coronary artery disease. *Prostaglandins, Leukotrienes and Essential Fatty Acids, 56*(5), 379–384.

Borrelli, F., & Izzo, A. (2000). The plant kingdom as a source of anti-ulcer remedies. *Phytotherapy Research, 14*(8), 581–591.

Bown, D. (1995). *The Herb Society of America encyclopedia of herbs and their uses.* New York: Dorling Kindersley Publishing.

Braeckman, J. (1994). The extract of *Seronoa repens* in the treatment of BPH: A multicenter open study. *Current Therapeutic Research, 55*, 776–785.

Bratman, S., & Kroll, D. (2000). *The natural pharmacist: Your complete guide to illnesses and their natural remedies* (pp. 141–142). CA: Prima Publishing.

Brauning et al. (1992). (S. Coble & C. Hobbs, Trans.). *Echinacea purpura* radix for strengthening the immune response in flu-like infections. *Zefur Phytotherapie, 13*, 7–13.

Brevoort, P. (1996). The U.S. botanical market-An overview. *HerbalGram, 36*, 49–57.

Brinkeborn, R., Shah, D., Geissbuhler, S., & Degening, F. H. (1998). Echinaforce in the treatment of acute colds. *Schweiz Zeitschrift GansheitsMedzin, 10*, 26–29.

Brinker, F. (1998). *Herb contraindications and drug interactions.* (2nd ed). Sandy, Oregon: Eclectic Medical Publications.

Brody, J (1985). *Jane Brody's good food book.* New York: W.W. Norton & Co.

Brown, D. (1995). *An introduction to phytotherapy: The medical uses of 8 common herbs.* Connecticut: Keats.

Brown, D., & Yarnell, E. (1996). *Phytotherapy research compendium.* WA: Natural Product Research Consultants.

Bruneton, J. (1995). *Pharmacognosy, Phytochemistry, Medicinal Plants.* Paris: Lavoisier Publishing. Cited in: M. Blumenthal, A. Goldberg, & J. Brinckmann (Eds.). (2000). *Herbal Medicine Expanded Commission E Monographs* (pp. 379–384). Austin, Tex: American Botanical Council; Boston: Integrative Medicine Communications.

Buck, D., Nidorf, D., & Addino, J. (1994). Comparison of two topical preparations for the treatment of onychomycosis: *Melaleuca alternifolia* (tea tree) oil and clotrimazole. *Journal of Family Practice, 38*, 601–605.

Budzinski, J., Foster, B., Vanderhoek, S., & Arnason, J. (2000). An in vitro evaluation of human cytochrome p450 3A4 inhibition by selected commercial herbal extracts and tinctures. *Phytomedicine, 7*(4), 273–282.

Burkhard, P., Burkhardt, K., Haenggeli, C., & Landis, T. (1999). Plant-induced seizures: Reappearance of an old problem. *Journal of Neurology, 246*(8), 667–670.

Calabrese, C., & Preston, P.(1993). Reports of a double-blind, randomized, single-dose trial of a topical 2% escin gel versus placebo in the acute treatment of experimentally induced hematoma in volunteers. *Planta Medica, 59*, 394–397.

Calixto, J.B., Beirith, A., Ferreira, J., Santos, A. R., Filho, V. C., & Yunes, R. A. (2000). Naturally occurring antinociceptive substances from plants. *Phytotherapy Research, 14*(6), 401–418.

Caplan, R. (1989). The commodification of American health care. *Social Science and Medicine, 328*, 1139–1148.

Carlson, C. (July/August 2000). Turmeric the gold standard of spices. *Herbs for Health*, 60–64.

310

Carson, C., Cookson, B., Farrelly, H. D., & Riley, T. V. (1995). Susceptibility of methicillin-resistant *Staphylococcus aureus* to the essential oil of *Melaleuca alternifolia. Journal of Antimicrobial Chemotherapy, 35*, 421–424.

Carson, C., & Riley, T. (1995). Antimicrobial activity of the major components of the essential oil of *Melaleuca alternifolia. Journal of Applied Bacteriology, 78*, 264–269.

Cerny, A., &Schmid, K. (1999). Tolerability and efficacy of valerian/lemon balm in healthy volunteers (a double-blind, placebo-controlled, multicentre study). *Filoterapia, 70*, 221–228.

Cetaruk, E. W., and Aaron, C. K. (1994). Hazards of nonprescription medications. *Emergency Medicine Clinics of North America, 12*(2), 483–510.

Chadha, Y, et al. (Eds.) (1952–1988). *The wealth of India*, 11 volumes. New Delhi: Publications and Information Directorate, CSIR. Cited in M. McGuffin, C. Hobbs, R. Upton, & A. Goldberg.(1997). *Botanical safety handbook* (p. 6). Boca Raton, FL: CRC Press.

Champault, G., Patel, J., & Bonnard, A. (1984). A double blind trial of an extract of the plant serenoa repens in BPH. *British Journal of Clinical Pharmacology, 18*, 461–462.

Chang, R. (1996). Functional properties of edible mushrooms. *Nutrition Review, 54*(11, Pt. 2), S91–S93.

Chatterjee, S., Bhattacharya, S., Wonnemann, M., et al. (1998). Hyperforin as a possible antidepressant component of *Hypericum* extracts. *Life Sciences, 63*(6), 499–510.

Chichon, P. (August 2000). Herbs and the common cold. *Advance for Nurse Practitioners*, 31–32.

Chrubasik, S., et al. (1997). Evidence for antirheumatic effectiveness of *Herba urticae dioicae* in acute arthritis: A pilot study. *Phytomedicine, 4*(2), 105–108.

Clinics of North America, 12, 497–510.

Collier, H., Butt, N., McDonald-Gibson, & Saeed, S. (October 25, 1980). Extract of feverfew inhibits prostaglandin biosynthesis. *The Lancet, 2*(8200), 922–923.

Craig WJ. (1999). Health-promoting properties of common herbs. *American Journal of Clinical Nutrition. 70*(3), 491S–499S.

Craig, WJ. (1997). Phytochemicals: Guardians of our health. *Journal of the American Diet Association, 10* (Suppl 2), S199–204.

Currier, N. L., & Miller, S. C. (2001). *Echinacea purpurea* and melatonin augment natural-killer cells in leukemic mice and prolong life span. *Journal of Alternative and Complementary Medicine, 7*(3), 241–251.

D'Angelo, L., Grimaldi, R., Caravaggi, M., Marcoli, M., Perucea, E., Lecchini, S., Frigo, G. M., & Crema, A. A double-blind, placebo controlled clinical study on the effect of a standardized ginseng extract on psychomotor performance in healthy volunteers. *Journal of Ethnopharmacology, 16*, 15–22.

Darlington, L. G., & Stone, T. W. (2001). Antioxidants and fatty acids in the amelioration of rheumatoid arthritis and related disorders. *The British Journal of Nutrition, 85*(3), 251–269.

Davis, R., DiDonato, J., Hartman, G., & Haas, R. (1994). Anti-inflammatory and wound healing activity of a growth substance in *Aloe vera. Journal of the American Podiatric Medical Association, 84*, 77–81.

Davis, R., DiDonato, J., Johnson, R., & Stewart, C. (1994). *Aloe vera*, hydrocortisone, and sterol influence on wound tensile strength and anti-inflammation. *Journal of the American Podiatric Medical Association, 84*, 614–621.

Davis, R., Stewart, G., & Bregman, P. (1992). Aloe vera and the inflamed synovial pouch model. *Journal of the American Podiatric Medical Association, 82*, 140–148.

DeClercq, E. (2000). Current lead natural products for the chemotherapy of human immunodeficiency virus (HIV) infection. *Medicinal Research Reviews, 20*(5), 323–49.

DeFeudis, F. V., & Drieu, K. (2000). Ginkgo biloba extract (Egb 761) and CNS functions: Basic studies and clinical applications. *Current Drug Targets, 1*(1), 25–28.

DeJesus, R., et al. (2000). Analysis of the antinociceptive properties of marrubiin isolated from *Marrubiim vulgare. Phytomedicine, 7*(2), 111–115.

De Leo, V., La Marca, A., Lanzetta, D., Palazzi, S., Torricelli, M., Facchini, C., & Morgante, G. (2000). Assessment of the association of kava-kava extract and hormone replacement therapy in the treatment of postmenopause anxiety [in Italian]. *Minerva Ginecologica* (*Torino*), *52*(6), 263–267.

DeLorgeril, M., et al. (1994). Mediterranean alpha-linolenic acid-rich diet in secondary prevention of coronary heart disease. *The Lancet, 343*, 1454–1459.

Dentali, S. (1997). HRF produces safety review on kava for AHPA. *HerbalGram, 40*, 14.

DeSmet, D., & D'Arcy, P.(1996). Drug interactions with herbal and other non-orthodox remedies. In:

P. D'Arcy, J. McElnay, & P. Welling (Eds.). *Mechanisms of drug interactions.* New York: Springer-Verlag 327–352.

Diehm, C., Trampisch, J., Lange, S., & Schmidt, C. (1996). Comparison of leg compression stocking and oral horse-chestnut seed extract therapy in patients with chronic venous insufficiency. *The Lancet, 347,* 292–294.

DiSilverio, F., et al. (1992). Evidence that *Serenoa repens* extract displays an antiestrogenic activity in prostatic tissue of BPH. *European Urology, 21,* 309–314.

Dixon-Shanties, D., & Shaikh, N. (1999). Growth inhibition of human breast cancer cells by herbs and phytoestrogens. *Oncology Reports, 6*(6), 1383–1387.

Djuric, Z., & Powell, L. C. (2001). Antioxidant capacity of lycopene-containing foods. *International Journal of Food Sciences and Nutrition, 52*(2), 143–149.

Dobbins, K., & Saul, R. (2000) Transient visual loss after licorice ingestion. *J Neuroopthalmology, 20*(1), 38–41.

Donath, F., Quispe, S., Diefenbach, K., Maurer, A., Fietze, I., and Roots, I. (2000). Critical evaluation of the effect of valerian extract on sleep structure and sleep quality. *Pharmacopsychiatry, 33*(2), 47–53.

Duke, J. (2000) Phytochemical and Ethnobotanical Database at the Agricultural Research Services. http://www.ars-grin.gov/duke/

Duker, E., Kopanski, L., Jarry, H., & Wuttke, W. (1991). Effects of extracts from Cimicifuga racemosa on gonadotropin release in menopausal women and ovariectomized rats. *Planta Medica, 57,* 420–424.

Eftekhar, J. (1996). *Garlic: The miracle herb.* FL: Globe Press.

Einer-Jensen, N., Zhao, J., Andersen, K., & Kristoffersen, K. (1996). *Cimicifuga* and *Melbrosia* lack oestrogenic effects in mice and rats. *Maturitas, 25,* 149–153.

Eisenberg, D. M., Davis, R. B., Ettner, S. L., Appel, S., Wilkey, S., Van Rompay, M., & Kessler, R. C. (1998). Trends in alternative medicine use in the United States, 1990–1997. *Journal of the American Medical Association, 280,* 1569–1575.

Eisenberg, D. M., Kessler, R. C., Foster, C., Norlock, F. E., Calkins, D. R., & Delbanco, T. L. (1993). Unconventional medicine in the United States. *New England Journal of Medicine, 328,* 246–252.

Engebretson, J., & Wardell, D. (September 1993). A contemporary view of alternative healing modalities. *Nurse Practitioner,* 51–55.

Ernst, E. (1997). Can allium vegetables prevent cancer? *Phytomedicine, 4*(1), 79–83.

Ernst, E., & Huntley, A. (2000). Tea tree oil: A systematic review of randomized clinical trials. *Forschende Komplementarmedizin und Klassische Naturheilkunde [Research in Complementary and Natural Classical Medicine), 7*(1), 17–20.

Ernst, E., & Pittler, M. H. (2000). The efficacy and safety of feverfew (*Tanacetum parthenium L.):* An update of a systemic review. *Public Health Nutrition, 3*(4A), 509–514

European Scientific Cooperative on Phytotherapy (ESCOP). (1999). *ESCOP monographs on the medicinal uses of plant drugs.* Exeter, UK: ESCOP.

Farese, R. V., Jr., Biglieri, E. G., Shackleton, C. H., Irony, I., & Gomez-Fontes, R. (1991). Licorice-induced hypermineralocorticoidism. *New England Journal of Medicine, 325*(17), 1223–1227.

Farnsworth, N., Akerele, O., Bingel, A. S., Soejarto, D. D., & Guo, Z. (1985). Medicinal plants in therapy. *Bulletin of the World Health Organization, 63*(6),39–31.

Fintelmann, V. (1986). Toxic metabolic liver damage and its treatment. *Zeitschrift fur Phytotherapie, 3,* 65–73.

Fisher-Rasmussen, W., Kjaer, S., Ddahl, C., & Asping, U. (1990). Ginger treatment of hyperemesis gravidarum. *Euopean Journal of Obstetrics, Gynecology, and Reproductive Biology, 38,* 19–24.

Ferrara, L., Montesano, D., & Senatore, A. (2001). The distribution of minerals and flavonoids in the tea plant (*Camillia sinensis*). *Farmaco, 56*(5–7), 397401.

Foo, L.Y., Lu, Y., Howell, A. B., & Vorsa, N (2000). The structure of cranberry proanthocyanidins which inhibit adherence of uropathogenic P-fimbriated *Escherichia coli* in vitro. *Phytochemistry, 54*(2), 173–81.

Food and Drug Administration (October 1983). Unsafe Herbs. *FDA Consumer.* [on line], Available: Hostname: http://lep.cl.msu.edu/msueimp/htdoc/modO3/03900066.html.

Ford, I., Cotter, M. A., Cameron, N. E., and Greaves, M. (2001). The effects of treatment with alpha-lipoic acid or evening primrose oil on vascular hemostatic and lipid risk factors, streptozotocin-diabetic rat. *Metabolism, 50*(8), 868–875.

312

Foster, S. (May/June 1999). Stress less. *Herbs for Health,* 38–42.

Foster, S. (1999). Black cohosh: A literature review. *HerbalGram, 45,* 35–49.

Foster, S. (January/February 2000). The latest on echinacea. *Herbs for Health,* 8–9.

Foster, S. (1998). *101 medicinal herbs.* Loveland, CO: Interweave Press.

Foster, S. (March 1996). Ginkgo biloba. *Herbs for Health,* 30–33.

Foster, S., & Duke, J. (1990). *Eastern/central medicinal plants.* New York: Houghton Mifflin.

Fox, H. (1953.) *The Years in My Herb Garden* (p. 116). New York: Macmillan Company.

French, M. (July 1996). The power of plants. *Advance for Nurse Practitioners,* 16–21.

French, M. (July 1996). The mind-body-spirit connection: An introduction to alternative therapies. *Advance for Nurse Practitioners,* 38–46.

Fugh-Berman, A. (September 6–13, 1993). The case for "natural" medicine. *The Nation,* 240–244.

Fugh-Berman, A. (May 13–17, 1996). Herb-drug interactions. Symposium conducted at the meeting of the Botanical Medicine in Modern Clinical Practice, Columbia University, NY, 143–156.

Fujisawa, Y., Sakamoto, M., Matsushita, M., Fujita, T., & Nishioka, K. (2000). Glycyrrhizin inhibits the lytic pathway of complement-possible mechanism of its anti-inflammatory effect on liver cells in viral hepatitis. *Microbiology and Immunology, 44*(9), 799–804.

Fukushima, M., Ohhashi, T., Ohno, S., Saitoh, H., Sonoyama, K., Shimada, K., Sekekawa, M., & Nakano, M. (2001).Effects of diets enriched in n-6 or n-3 fatty acids on cholesterol metabolism in older rats chronically fed a cholesterol-enriched diet. *Lipids, 36*(3), 261–266.

Fussel, A., Wolf, A., & Brattstrom, A. (2000). Effect of a fixed valerian-hop extract combination (Ze91019) on sleep polygraphy in patients with non-organic insomnia: A pilot study. *European Journal of Medical Research, 5*(9), 385–390.

Garg, S., & Sharma, S. N. (1992). Development of medicated aerosol dressings of chlorhexidine acetate with hemostatics. *Pharmazie, 47*(12), 924–926.

Giovannucci, E., Ascherio, A., Rimm, E. B., et al. (1995). Intake of carotenoids and retinol in relation to risk of prostate cancer. *Journal of National Cancer Institute, 87,* 1767–1776.

Gollapudi, S., Sharma, H. A., Aggarwal, S., Byers, L. D., Ensley, H. E., & Gupta, S. (1995). Isolation of a previously unidentified polysaccharide (MAR 10) from *Hyssop officinalis* that exhibits strong activity against human immunodeficiency virus type 1. *Biochemical and Biophysical Research Communications, 210*(1), 145–151.

Govindan, M., & Govindan, G. (2000). A convenient method for the determination of the quality of goldenseal. *Fitoterapia, 71*(3), 232–235.

Graf, J. (2000). Herbal anti-inflammatory agents for skin disease. *Skin Therapy Letter, 5*(4), 3–5.

Griggs, B. (1981). *Green pharmacy: The history and evolution of western herbal medicine.* VT: Healing Arts Press.

Guthrie, D. (August 2000). Herbal approaches to diabetes care. *Advance for Nurse Practitioners,* 56–59.

Haggerty, W. Flax: Ancient herb and modern medicine. *HerbalGram, 45,* 51–57.

Hallstrom, C., Fulder, S., & Carruthers, M. (1982). Effect of ginseng on the performance of nurses on night duty. *Complementary Medicine East and West, 6,* 277–282.

Hanak, T., & Bruckel, M. (1983). Treatment of moderately stable forms of angina pectoris with *Crataegutt novo* [in German]. *Therapiewoche, 33,* 4331–4333.

Hardy, M. L. (2000). Herbs of special interest to women. *Journal of the American Pharmaceutical Association, 40*(2), 234–242.

Hasler, C. M., Kundtat, S., & Wool, D. (2000). Functional foods and cardiovascular disease. *Current Atherosclerosis Reports, 2*(6), 467–475.

Harrer, G., & Schulz, V. (1994). Clinical investigation of the antidepressant effectiveness of hypericum. *Journal of Geriatric Psychiatry and Neurology, 7,* S6–S8.

Hatano, T., et al. (2000). Phenolic constituents of licorice.VIII. Structures of glicophenone and glico and effects of licorice phenolics on methicillin resistant *Staphylococcus aureus. Chemical and Pharmaceutical Bulletin (Tokyo), 48*(9), 1286–1292.

Heck, A., Dewitt, B., & Lukes, A. (2000). Potential interactions between alternative therapies and warfarin. *American Journal of Health-System Pharmacy, 57*(13), 1221–1227.

Heptinstall, S., Awang, D. V., Dawson, B. A., Kindack, D., Knight, D. W., & May, J. (1992). Parthenolide content and bioactivity of feverfew. Estimation of commercial and authenticated feverfew products. *Journal of Pharmacy and Pharmacology, 44*(5), 390–395.

313

Heptinstall, S., Williamson, L., White, A., & Mitchell, J. (May 11, 1985). Extracts of feverfew inhibit granule secretion in blood platelets and polymorphonuclear leucocytes. *The Lancet,* 1071–1073.

HerbalGram (1999). No. 46.

Herb Research News. (1996, Fall). Newsletter.

Herbst, D. (September 1999.). Bad mix. *Natural Health,* 100–103, 147.

Ho, S. C., Chan, S. G., Yi, Q., Wong, E., & Leung, P. C. (2001). Soy intake and the maintenance of peak bone mass in Hong Kong Chinese women. *Journal of Bone and Mineral Research, 16*(7), 1363–1369.

Hobbs, C. (January/February 2000). Cancer-fighting mushrooms. *Herbs for Health,* 59–60.

Hobbs, C. (1994). Echinacea: A literature review. *HerbalGram,* 30.

Hofferberth, B. (1994). The efficacy of EGb 761 in patients with senile dementia of the Alzheimer type, a double-blind, placebo-controlled study on different levels of investigation. *Human Psychopharmacology, 9,* 215–222.

Hoffman, D. (1994). *The information sourcebook of herbal medicine.* Freedom, CA: The Crossing Press.

Hoffman, D. (1992). *The new holistic herbal.* Boston, MA: Element.

Holt, S. (1997). Phytoestrogens for a healthier menopause. *Alternative and Complementary Therapies, 3*(3), 187–193.

Holt, S., Muntyan, I., & Likver, L. (1996). Soya-based diets for diabetes mellitus. *Alternative and Complementary Therapies, 2*(2), 79–82.

Holtmann, S., Clarke, A., Scherer, H., & Hohn, M. (1989). The anti-motion sickness mechanism of ginger. *Acta Oto-Laryngologica, 108,* 168–174.

Horn-Ross, P., Barnes, S., Lee, M., Coward, L., Mandel, J., Koo, J., John, E, & Smith, M. (2000). Assessing phytoestrogen exposure in epidemiologic studies: development of a database. *Cancer Causes Control, 11*(4), 289–298.

Horrobin, D. .F. (2000). Essential fatty acid metabolism and its modification in atopic eczema. *American Journal of Nutrition, 71*(1 Suppl), 367S–372S.

Hou, J. P. (1977). The chemical constituents of ginseng plants. *Complementary Medicine East and West, 5*(2), 123–145.

Howell, A. B., Vorsa, N., Der Marderosian, A., & Foo Ly. (1998). Inhibition of the adherence of p-fimbriated *Escherichia coli* to uroepithelial-cell surfaces by proanthocyanidin extracts from cranberries. *New England Journal of Medicine, 339*(15), 1085–1086.

Hubner, W. D., & Kirste, T. (2001). Experience with St. John's wort (*Hypericum perforatum*) in children under 12 years with symptoms of depression and psychovegetative disturbances. *Phytotherapy Research, 15*(4), 367–370.

Hulley, S., Grady, D., Bush, T., Furberg, C., Herrington, D., Riggs, B., & Vittinghoff, E. (1998). Randomized trial of estrogen plus progestin for secondary prevention of coronary heart disease in postmenopausal women. *Journal of the American Medical Association, 280,* 605–613.

Imai, K., & Nakachi, K. (1995). Cross sectional study of effects of drinking green tea on cardiovascular and liver diseases. *British Medical Journal, 310,* 693–696.

International Journal of Cancer, 70(6), 669–705.

Israelson, L., & Blumenthal, M. (2000). FDA issues final rules for structure/function claims for dietary supplements. *HerbalGram,* 48, 32–38.

Jain, N. K., & Kulkarni, S. K. (1999). Antinociceptive and anti-inflammatory effects of *Tanacetum parthenium L.* extract in mice and rats. *Journal of Ethnopharmacology, 68*(1–3), 251–259.

Johnson, E., Kadam, N., Hylands, D., & Hylands, P. (1985). Efficacy of feverfew as prophylactic treatment of migraine. *British Medical Journal, 291,* 569–573.

Jones, D. L., Kroenke, K., Landry, F. J., Tomich, D. J., & Ferrel, R. J. (1996). Cost savings using a stepped-care prescribing protocol for nonsteroidal anti-inflammatory drugs. *Journal of the American Medical Association, 275*(12), 926–930.

Joshi, S. S., Kuszynski, C. A., & Bagchi, D. (2001). The cellular and molecular basis of health benefits of grape seed proanthocyanidin extract. *Current Pharmaceutical Biotechnology, 2*(2), 187–200.

Kabir, Y., & Kimura, S. (1989). Dietary mushrooms reduce blood pressure in spontaneously hypertensive rats (SHR). *Journal of Nutritional Science and Vitaminology (Tokyo), 35*(1), 91–94.

Kalvatchev, Z., Walder, R., & Garzaro, D. (1997). Anti-HIV activity of extracts from *Calendula officinalis* flowers. *Biomedicine and Pharmacotherapy, 51*(4), 176–180.

Kane, S., & Goldberg, M. (2000) Use of bromelain in the treatment of mild ulcerative colitis. *Annals of Internal Medicine, 132*(8), 680.

Kannar, D., Wattanapenpaiboon, D., Savige, G. S., & Walhquist, M. L. (2001). Hypocholesteremic effect of an enteric-coated garlic supplement. *Journal of American College of Nutrition, 20*(3), 225–231.

Kanowski, D., Herrmann, W. M., Stephan, K., Wierich, W., & Horr, R. (1996). Proof of efficacy of the *Ginkgo biloba* special extract Egb 761 in outpatients suffering from mild to moderate primary degenerative dementia of the Alzheimer type or multi-infarct dementia. *Pharmacopsychiatry, 29,* 47–56.

Katiyar, S., Agarwal, R., & Mukhatar, H. (1992). Green tea in chemoprevention of cancer. *Comprehensive Therapy, 18*(10), 3–8.

Keen, H, Payan, J., Allawi, J., Waslker, J., Jamal, G. A., Weir, A. I., Henderson, L. M., Bissessar, E. A., Watkins, P. J., Sampson, M., et al. (1993). Treatment of diabetic neuropathy with gamma-linolenic acid. *Diabetes Care, 16*(1), 8–15.

Kettler, D. B. (2001). Can manipulation of the ratios of essential fatty acids slow the rapid rate of postmenopausal bone loss? *Alternative Medicine Review, 6*(1), 61–77.

Khalsa, K. (September/October 2000). Red raspberries may prevent cancer. *Herbs for Health,* 16.

Kleinjen, J., & Knipschild, P. (1992). Ginkgo biloba. *The Lancet, 340,* 1136–1139.

Klepser, T. B., & Klepser, M. E. (1999). Unsafe and potentially safe herbal therapies. *American Journal of Health-System Pharmacology, 56*(2), 125–138.

Klepser, T., & Nisly, N. (June 1999). Chaste tree berry for premenstrual syndrome. *Alternative Medicine Alert,* 63–66.

Kline, R. M., Kline, J. J., Di Palma, J., & Barbero, G. J. (2001). Enteric-coated, pH-dependent peppermint oil capsules for the treatment of irritable bowel syndrome in children. *Journal of Pediatrics, 138*(1), 125–128.

Knight, J. (November/December 2000). Soy meets world. *Herbs for Health,* 39–44.

Knoben, J., & Anderson, P. (1993). *Handbook of clinical drug data* (pp. 626–627). IL: Drug Intelligence Publications.

Kontiokari, T., Sundqvist, K., Nuutinen, M., Pokka, T., & Uhari, M. (2001). Randomised trial of cranberry-lingonberry juice and lactobacillus GG drink for the prevention of urinary tract infections in women. *British Medical Journal, 322*(7302), 1571.

Koscielny, J, et al. (1999). The antiatherosclerotic effect of *Allium sativum. Artherosclerosis, 144,* 237–249.

Kowalchik C., & Hylton, W. (eds.). (1987). *Rodale's illustrated encyclopedia of herbs.* Emmaus, PA: Rodale Press.

Kreus, W., et al. (1990). Inhibition of HIV replication by *Hyssop officinalis* extracts. *Antiviral Research, 14*(6), 323–337.

Kubo, K., & Nanba, H. (1996). The effect of maitake mushrooms on liver and serum lipids. *Alternative Therapies in Health and Medicine, 2*(5), 62–66.

Kuhn, M. (1999). Letter. *Complementary Therapy-Gram* 2(1).

Lacomblez, L., Bensimon, G., Isnard, F., Diquet, B., Lecrubier, Y., & Puech, A. J. (March 1989). Effect of yohimbine on blood pressure in patients with depression and orthostatic hypertension induced by clomipramine. *Clinical and Pharmacological Therapeutics, 45,* 241–251. Cited in *HerbalGram, 49,* 62.

Ladanyi, A., Timar, J., & Lapis, K. (1993). Effect of Lentinan on macrophage cytoxicity against metastatic tumor cells. *Cancer Immunology, Immunotherapy, 36,* 123–6.[Medline]

Lantz, M., Buchalter, E., & Giambanco, V. (1999). St. John's wort and antidepressant drug interactions in the elderly. *Journal of Geriatric Psychiatry and Neurology, 12,* 7–10.

Lauritzen, C., et al. (1997). Treatment of premenstual tension syndrome with *Vitex agnus-castus.* Controlled, double-blind study versus pyrodoxine. *Phytomedicine, 4*(3), 183–189.

Lawless, J. (1997). *The complete illustrated guide to aromatherapy.* MA: Element, Inc.

Lawrence Review of Natural Products (1994). Feverfew. Facts and Comparisons. St. Louis, MO.

Lawson, L. D., Wang, Z. J., & Papadimitriou, D. (2001). Allicin release under simulated gastrointestinal conditions from garlic powder tablets employed in clinical trials on serum cholesterol. *Planta Medica, 67*(1), 13–18.

Leathwood, P., Chafford, F., Heck, E., & Munoz-Box, R. (1982). Aqueous extract of valerian root (*Valeriana officinalis L.*) improves sleep quality in man. *Pharmacology, Biochemistry and Behavior, 17,* 65–71.

LeBars, P. L., & Kastelan, J. (2000). Efficacy and safety of a *Ginkgo biloba* extract. *Public Health Nutrition, 3*(4A), 495–499.

Lenoir, S., Degenring, F., & Saller, R.(1999). A double-blind randomized trial to investigate three different concentrations of a standardized fresh plant extract obtained from the shoot tips of *Hypericum perforatum L. Phytomedicine, 6*(3), 141–146.

Leung, A. (1980). *Encyclopedia of common natural ingredients used in foods, drugs and cosmetics* (pp. 74–76). New York: John Wiley & Sons.

Levy, A. M., Kita, H., Phillips, S. F., Schnade, P. A., Dyer, P. D., Gleich, G. J., & Dubravec, V. A. (1998). Eosinophilia and gastrointestinal symptoms after ingestion of shiitake mushrooms. *Journal of Allergy and Clinical Immunology, 101*(5), 613–620.

Le Bars, P. (1997). A placebo-controlled, double-blind, randomized trial of an extract of Ginkgo biloba for dementia. *Journal of the American Medical Association, 278*(16), 1327–1332.

Lieberman, S. (1998). A review of the effectiveness of *Cimicifuga racemosa* (black cohosh) for the symptoms of menopause. *Journal of Women's Health, 7*(5), 525–529.

Lindahl, O., & Lindwall, L. (1989). Double blind study of a valerian preparation. *Pharmacology, Biochemistry and Behavior, 32*(4),1065–1066.

Linde, K., & Mulrow, C. (1999). St. John's wort for depression. In *The Cochrane Library,* Issue 4, 1998. Oxford. Cited in *The integrative medicine consult* (February 1, 1999).

Lindenmuth, G. F., & Lindenmuth, E. B. (2000). The efficacy of echinacea compound herbal tea preparation on the severity and duration of upper respiratory and flu symptoms: A randomized, double-blind placebo-controlled study. *Journal of Alternative and Complementary Medicine, 6*(4), 327–334.

Liske, E. (1998). Therapeutic efficacy and safety of *Cimicifuga racemosa* for gynecologic disorders. *Advances in Therapy, 15*(1), 45–53.

Liu, Z., Yang, Z., Zhu, M., & Huo, J. (2001). Estrogenicity of black cohosh (*Cimicifuga racemosa*) and its effect on estrogen receptor level in human breast cancer MCF-7 cells. *Wei Sheng Yan Jiu [Journal of Hygiene Research], 30*(2), 77-80.

Loch, E.G., Selle, H., & Boblitz, N. (2000). Treatment of premenstrual syndrome with a phytopharmaceutical formulation containing *Vitex agnus castus. Journal of Womens Health Gender-Based Medicine, 9*(3), 315–320.

Love, L. (1998). The MedWatch Program. *Clinical Toxicology, 36,* 263–267.

Lu, L. J., Anderson, K. E., Grady, J. J., & Nagamani, M. (2001). Effects of an isoflavone-free soy diet on ovarian hormones in premenopausal women. *The Journal of Clinical Endocrinology and Metabolism, 86*(7), 3045–3052.

Lumb, A. (1994). Effect of ginger on human platelet function. *Thrombosis and Haemostasis, 71,* 110–111. Cited in *HerbalGram, 49,* 60.

Lyon, M. R., Cline, J. C., Totosy de Zepetnek, J., Shan, J. J., Pang, P., & Benishin, C. (2001). Effect of the herbal extract combination *Panax quinquefolium* and *Ginkgo biloba* on attention-deficit hyperactivity disorder: A pilot study. *Journal of Psychiatry and Neuroscience, 26*(3), 221–228.

Makheja, A., Bailey, L. (November 7, 1981). The active principle in feverfew. *The Lancet,* 1054.

Mark, J. D., Grant, K. L., & Barton, L. L. (2001). The use of dietary supplements in pediatrics: A study of echinacea. *Clinical Pediatrics, 40*(5):265–269.

Marks, L. S., Partin, A. W., Epstein, J. I., Tyler, V. E., Simon, I., Macairan, M. L., Chan, T. L., Dorey, F. J., Garris, J. B., Veltri, R. W., Santos, P. B., Stonebrook, K. A., & de Kernion, J. B. (2000). Effects of a saw palmetto herbal blend in men with symptomatic benign prostatic hyperplasia. *Journal of Urology, 163*(5), 1451–1456.

Marles, R., & Farnsworth, N. (1995). Antidiabetic plants and their active constituents. *Phytomedicine, 2*(2), 137–189.

Marwick, C. (1995). Growing use of medicinal botanicals forces assessmnt by drug regulators. *Journal of the American Medical Association, 273*(8), 607–609.

May, B., Kohler, S., & Schneider, B. (2000). Efficacy and tolerability of a fixed combination of peppermint oil and caraway oil in patients suffering from functional dyspepsia. *Alimentary Pharmacology and Therapeutics, 14*(12), 1671–1677.

Mayell, M. (2001). Maitake extracts and their therapeutic potential. *Alternative Medicine Review, 6*(1), 48–60.

McCaleb, R. (March 1996). Herbal help for prostate problems. *Herbs for Health,* 27–28.

McCaleb, R. (1996, May 13–17). Herbal product sources and resources; Herbal product assessment. Symposium conducted at the meeting of the Botanical Medicine in Modern Clinical Practice, Columbia University, NY.

McCaleb, R. (May 25, 1993). Herb safety report. *Herb Research Foundation,* 1–4.

McCaleb, R., & Blumenthal. M. (1997). Research reviews. *HerbalGram,* 24–26.

McCaleb, R., Leigh, E., & Morien, K. (2000). *The encyclopedia of popular herbs.* Roseville, CA: Prima Publishing.

McFarlin, B., Gibson, M., O'Rear, J., & Harmon, P.(May–June 1999). A national survey of herbal preparation use by nurse-midwives for labor stimulation: review of the literature and recommendations for practice. *Journal of Nurse Midwifery, 44*(3), 183–188, 205–216.

McGuffin, M. (2000). Self regulatory initiatives by the herbal industry. *HerbalGram, 48,* 42–43.

McGuffin, M., Hobbs, C., Upton, R., & Goldberg, A. (1997). *Botanical safety handbook.* Boca Raton, FL: CRC Press.

Mennini, T., et al. (1993). In vitro study on the interaction of extracts and pure compounds from *Valeriana officinalis* roots with GABA, benzodiazepine and barbiturate receptors in rat brain. *Filoterapia, 54,* 291–300.

Michelfield, G., Grieving, I., & May, B. (2000). Effects of peppermint oil and caraway oil on gastroduodenal motility. *Phytotherapy Research, 14*(1), 20–23.

Miller, L. (1998). Herbal medicinals: Selected clinical considerations focusing on known or potential drug-herb interactions. *Archives of Internal Medicine, 158,* 2200–2211. Cited in Vickers & Zollman (1999). Herbal medicine. *British Medical Journal, 319,* 1050–1053.

Mizuno, T. (1995). *Shiitake Lentinus edodes:* Functional properties for medicinal and food purposes. *Food Review International, 11,* 111–128.

Mohrig, A., & Alken, R. (1996). Meta-analysis of a placebo-controlled clinical trial of Lomaherpan treatment in Herpes simplex at various locations. Berlin.

Morien, K. (Summer, 1998). Kava (*Piper methysticum*). Newsletter. *Herb Research Foundation,* 4–5.

Morelli, V., & Zoorob, R. J. (2000). Alternative therapies: Part II. Congestive heart failure and hypercholesterolemia. *American Family Physician, 62*(6), 1325–1330.

Mouren, X., Caillard, P., & Schwartz, F. (1994). Study of the anti-ischemic action of Egb761 in the treatment of peripheral arterial occlusive disease by TcPO2 determination. *Angiology, 45,* 413–417.

Mowrey, D., & Clayson, D. (March 20, 1982). Motion sickness, ginger, and psychophysics. *The Lancet,* 655–657.

Mukhatar, H., Wang, Z., & Katiyar, S. (1992). Tea components: Antimutagenic and anticarcinogenic effects. *Preventive Medicine, 21,* 351–360.

Mullins, R. (1998). Echinacea-associated anaphylaxis. *Medical Journal of Australia, 16*(4), 170–171.

Murphy, J., Heptinstall, S., & Mitchell, J. (July 23, 1988). Randomized double-blind placebo-controlled trial of feverfew in migraine prevention. *The Lancet,* 189–192.

Murray, M. (1995). *The Healing Power of Herbs.* Roseville, CA: Prima Publishing.

Murray, M., & Werbach, M. (1994). *Botanical Influences on Illness.* Tarzana, CA: Third Line Press.

Murray, M. A natural alternative to estrogen for menopause. *Cimicifuga* extract (Black cohosh). *Health Counselor, 8,* 36–37.

Nagabhushan, N., & Bhide, S. (1992). Curcumin as an inhibitor of cancer. *Journal of the American College of Nutrition, 11,* 192–198.

Nanba, H. (February/March 1996). Maitake D-fraction healing and preventing potentials for cancer. *Townsend Letter for Doctors and Patients,* 84–85.

Natural Medicines Comprehensive Database. (2000). *Pharmacist's Letter and Prescriber's Letter.* Therapeutic Research Faculty.

Negro, A., Rossi, E., Regolisti, G., & Perazzoli, F. (2000). Liquorice-induced sodium retention. Merely an acquired condition of apparent mineralocorticoid excess? A case report. *Annali Italiani di Medicina Interna: Organo Ufficiale della Società Italiana di Medicina Interna, 15*(4), 296–300.

Neurauer, R. (1961). A plant protease for potentiation of and possible replacement of antibiotics. *Experimental Medicine and Surgery, 19,* 143–160. Cited in HerbalGram, *49,* 58.

317

Ody, P. (1993). *The complete medicinal herbal.* New York: Dorling Kindersley Publishing.

Olukoga A., & Donaldson, D. (2000) Liquorice and its health implications. *Journal of the Royal Society of Health, 120*(2), 83–89.

Onning, G., Wallmark, A., Persson, M., Akesson, B., Elm Stahl, S., & Oste, R. (1999). Consumption of oat milk for 5 weeks lowers serum cholesterol and LDL cholesterol in free-living men with moderate hyper-cholesterolemia. *Annals of Nutrition and Metabolism, 43*(5), 301–309.

Orekhov, A., Tertov, V., Sobenin, I., & Pivovarova, E. (1994). Direct anti-atherosclerosis related effects of garlic. *Annals of Medicine, 27,* 63–65.

Ottariano, S. (1999). *Medicinal herbal therapy: A pharmacist's viewpoint.* North Hampton, NH: Nicolin Fields Publishing.

Overmyer, M. (1999). Saw palmetto shown to shrink prostatic epithelium. *Urology Times, 27*(6), 1, 42.

Palasciano, G., et al. (1994). The effect of silymarin on plasma levels of malon-dialdehyde in patients receiving long-term treatment with psychotropic drugs. *Current Therapeutic Research, 55,* 537–545.

Palevitch, D., Earon. G., & Carosso, R. (1997). Feverfew (*Tanacetum parthenium*) as a prophylactic treatment for migraine: a double-blind-placebo-controlled study. *Phytotherapy Research, 2,* 508–511.

Parbtani, A., & Clark (1996). Chapter 17: Flaxseed and its components in renal disease. In *Flaxseed in Human Nutrition* (*p. 244*). ILL:AOCS Press. Cited in W. Haggerty. Flax, ancient herb and modern medicine. *HerbalGram, 45,* 54–55.

Park, H., Rhee, M. H., Park, K. M., Nam, K. Y., & Park, K. H. (1995). Effect of non-saponin fraction from *Panax ginseng* on cGMP and thromboxane A2 in human platelet aggregation. *Journal of Ethnopharmacology, 49,*157–62 [Medline].

Parnham, M. (1996). Benefit-risk assessment of the squeezed sap of the purple coneflower (*E. purpurea*) for long-term oral immunostimulation. *Phytomedicine, 3*(1), 95–102.

Patil, S. P., Niphadkar, P. V., & Bapat, M. M. (1997). Allergy to fenugreek (*Trigonella foenum graecom*). *Annals of Allergy, Asthma and Immunology, 78*(3), 297–300.

Patrick, K., Kumar, S., Edwardson, P., & Hutchinson, J. J. (1996). Induction of vascularisation by an aqueous extract of the flowers of *Calendula officinalis. Phytomedicine, 3,* 11–18.

PDR for herbal medicines (1998). Montvale, NJ: Medical Economics Company.

Pena, E. (1962). *Melaleuca alternifolia* oil. *Obstetrics and Gynecology, 19,* 793–795.

Piscitelli, S. C., Burstein, A. H., Chai, H. D., Alfaro, R. M., & Falloon, J. (2000). Indinavir concentrations and St. John's wort. *The Lancet, 355,* 547–548.

Pittler, M. H, & Ernst, E.(1998). Horse chestnut seed extract for chronic venous insufficiency: a criteria-based systematic review. *Archives of Dermatology, 134,* 1356–1360.

Pittler, M. H., & Ernst, E. (2000). Efficacy of kava extract for treating anxiety: Systematic review and meta-analysis. *Journal of Clinical Psychopharmacology, 20*(1), 84–89.

Pizzorno, J. (September–October 1996) 10 drugs I would never take. *Natural Health,* 84–88.

Potter, S. M., Baum, J. A., Teng, H., Stillman, R. J., Shay, N. F., & Erdman, J. W., Jr. (1998). Soy protein and isoflavones: Their effects on blood lipids and bone density in post-menopausal women. *American Journal of Clinical Nutrition, 68*(6 Suppl), 1375S–1379S.

Prasad, K. (2001). Secoisolariciresinol diglucoside (SDG) from flaxseed delays the development of type 2 diabetes in Zucker rat. *Journal of Laboratory and Clinical Medicine, 138*(1), 32–39.

Prescriber's Letter. (October 2000). Soy supplements, p. 58.

Prescriber's Letter. (September 2000). Neurology/psychiatry, p. 53.

Presidential commission reviews testimony on herbs and other natural products (Fall 1996). *Herb Research News,* 1–6.

Prevention Magazine (April/May1999). National Survey of Consumer Use of Dietary Supplements. Cited in *HerbalGram* (2000), *48,* 65.

Prucksunand, C., Indrasukhsri, B., Leethochawalit, M., & Hungspreugs, K. (2001). Phase II clinical trial on effect of the long turmeric (Curcuma longa Linn) on healing of peptic ulcer. *The Southeast Asian Journal of Tropical Medicine and Public Health, 32*(1), 208–215.

Rafi, M. (2000). Modulation of bcl-2 and cytotoxicity by licochalcone-A, a novel estrogenic flavonoid. *Anticancer Research, 20*(4), 2653–2658.

318

Ramsey, L., et al. (February 2000). Efficacy, safety, reliability: Common concerns about herbal products. *Advance for Nurse Practitioners, 31–33, 86.*

Rau, E. (2000). Treatment of acute tonsillitis with a fixed-combination herbal preparation. *Advances in Therapy, 17*(4), 197-203.

Richelle, M., Tavazzi, I., & Offord, E. (2001). Comparison of the antioxidant activity of commonly consumed polyphenolic beverages (coffee, cocoa, and tea) prepared per cup serving. *Journal of Agriculture and Food Chemistry, 49*(7), 3438–3442.

Ridker, P. M., & McDermott, W. V. (1989). Comfrey herb tea and hepatic veno-occlusive disease. *The Lancet, 1*(8639), 657–658.

Roberts, D., & Travis, E. (1995). Acemannan-containing wound dressing gel reduces radiation-induced skin reactions in C3H mice. *International Journal of Radiation Oncology, Biology, Physics, 32,* 1047–1052.

Roby, C. A., Anderson, G. D., Kantor, E., Dryer, D. A., & Burstein, A. H. (2000). St. John's wort: Effect on CYP3A4 activity. *Clinical Pharmacology and Therapeutics, 67,* 451–457.

Roman Ramos, R., Alarcon-Aguilar, F., Lara-Lemus, A., & Flores-Saenz, J. (1992, Spring). Hypoglycemic effect of plants used in Mexico as antidiabetics. *Archives of Medical Research, 23*(1), 59–64.

Romics, I., Schmitz, H., & Frang, D. (1993). Experience in treating benign prostatic hypertrophy with *Sabal serrulata* for one year. *International Urology and Nephrology, 25,* 565–569.

Roncin, J., Schwartz, F., & D'Arbigny, P. (1996). Egb 761 in control of acute mountain sickness and vascular reactivity to cold exposure. *Aviation Space and Environmental Medicine, 67*(5), 445–452.

Rosenblatt, M., & Mindel, J. (1997). Spontaneous hyphema associated with ingestion of Ginkgo biloba extract [letter]. *New England Journal of Medicine, 336*(15), 1108.

Rosso, J. (1993). *Great good food (p. 55).* New York: Crown.

Roundtree, R. (January 2001). Wishing you a safe New Year. *Herbs for Health,* 39–41.

Roundtree, R. (November/December 2000). Immune suppressants and herbal medicines. *Herbs for Health,* 26–27.

Ruschitzka, F., Meier, P. J., Turina, M., Luscher, T. F., & Noll, G.. Acute heart transplant rejection due to St. John's wort. *The Lancet, 355,* 548–549.

Saltzman, E., Das, K., Lichtenstein, A. H., Dallal, G. E., Corrales, A., Schaefer, E. J., Greenberg, A. S., & Roberts, S. B. (2001). An oat-containing hypocaloric diet reduces systolic blood pressure and improves lipid profile beyond effects of weight loss in men and women. *Journal of Nutrition, 131*(5), 1465–1470.

Sarrell, E. M., Mandelberg, A., & Cohen, H. A. (2001). Efficacy of naturopathic extracts in the management of ear pain associated with acute otitis media. *Archives of Pediatric and Adolescent Medicine, 155*(7), 796–799.

Schellenberg, R. (2001). Treatment for the premenstrual syndrome with *Agnus castus* fruit extract: Prospective, randomized, placebo controlled study. *British Medical Journal, 322*(7279), 134-137.

Schelosky, L., Raffauf, C., Jendroska, K., & Poewe, W. (1995). Kava and dopamine antagonism. *Journal of Neurology, Neurosurgery and Psychiatry, 58*(5), 639–640.

Schmidt, U., Kuhn, U., Ploch, M., et al. (1994). Efficacy of the Hawthorne (*Crataegus*) preparation LI 132 in 78 patients with chronic CHF defined as NYHA functional class II. *Phytomedicine, 1:*17–24.

Schneider,H., & Masuhr, T. (1995). Treatment of benign prostatic hyperplasia: Results of a surveillance study in the practices of urological specialists using a combined plant-based preparation. *Fortschritte der Medizin, 113:*37–40.

Schnitzler, P., Schon, K., & Reichling, J. (2001). Antiviral activity of Australian tea tree oil and eucalyptus oil against herpes simplex virus in cell culture. *Pharmazie, 56*(4), 343–347.

Schoneberger, D. (1992) (Sigrid & Klein, Trans.). The influence of immune stimulant effects of pressed juice from *Echinacea purpurea* on the course and severity of colds. *Forum Immunologie,* 2–12.

Schubert, H, & Halama, P. (1993). Depressive episode primarily unresponsive to therapy in elderly patients: Efficacy of *Ginkgo biloba* extract (Egb 761) in combination with antidepressants. *Geriatrie Forschrift, 3,* 45–53.

Scott, J.(1990). *Natural medicine for children.* London: Gaia.

Scrimal, R., & Dhawan, B. (1973). Pharmacology of diferuloyl methane (curcumin), a non-steroidal anti-inflammatory agent. *Journal of Pharmacy and Pharmacology, 25,* 447–452.

Shanmugasundaram, E., Rajeswari, G., Baskaran, K., Rajesh Kumar, B. R., Radha Shanmugasundaram, K., & Kizar Ahmath, B. (1990). Use of *Gymnema sylvestre* leaf extract in the control of blood glucose in insulin-dependent diabetes mellitus. *Journal of Ethnopharmacology, 30,* 281–294. Cited by F. Brinker (1998). *Herb contraindications and drug interactions.* (2nd ed). OR: *Eclectic Medical Publications.*

Sharma, R., Raghuram, T., & Rao, N. (1990). Effect of fenugreek seeds on blood glucose and serum lipids in type I diabetes. *European Journal of Clinical Nutrition, 44,* 301–306.

Sharma, R., Sarkar, A., Hazra, D., Misra, J., Singh, J., Maheshwari, B., & Sharma, S. (1996).Hypolipidaemic effect of fenugreek seeds: A chronic study in non-insulin dependent diabetic patients. *Phytotherapy Research, 10,* 332–334.

Shelton, R., et al. (2001). Effectiveness of St. John's wort in major depression. *Journal of the American Medical Association, 285,* 1978–1986.

Schrader, E. (2000). Equivalence of a St. John's wort extract (Ze 117) and fluoxetine: a randomized, controlled study in mild-moderate depression. *International Clinical Psychopharmacology, 15*(2), 61–68.

Shulman, A. (1997). Toxicological problems of traditional remedies and food supplements. *International Journal of Alternative and Complementary Medicine,* 9–10.

Sikora, R., Sohn, M., Deutz. F., et al. (1989). *Ginkgo biloba* extract in the therapy of erectile dysfunction [abstract]. *Journal of Urology, 141,* 188A.

Silagy, C., & Neil, A. (1993) A meta-analysis of the effect of garlic on blood pressure. *Journal of Hypertension, 12,* 463–468.

Silagy, C., & Neil, A. (1994). Garlic as a lipid lowering agent—A meta-analysis. *Journal of Royal College of Physicians London, 28,* 2–8.

Smith, H., Memon, A., Smart, C., & Dewbury, K.(1986).The value of Permixon in BPH. *British Journal of Urology, 58,* 36–40.

Smyth, R., Moss, J., Brennan, R., Harris, J., & Martin, G. (1967). Biochemical studies on the resolution of experimental inflammations in animals treated with bromelain. *Experimental Medicine and Surgery, 25,* 229–235.

Soller, W. Regulation in the Herb market: The myth of the "unregulated industry." *HerbalGram, 49,* 64–68.

Sommer. H., & Harrer, G. (1994). Placebo-controlled double-blind study examining the effectiveness of an *hypericum* preparation in 105 mildly depressed patients. *Journal of Geriatric Psychiatry and Neurology, 7,* S9–S11.

Sowmya, P, & Rajyalakshmi, P. (1999). Hypocholesterolemic effect of germinated fenugreek seeds in human subjects. *Plant Foods and Human Nutrition, 53*(4), 359–365.

Spencer Information Services (SPINS) Natural Track: AC Nielsen ScanTrack, SPINS Distributor Information.

Starr, P. (1982). *The social transformation of American medicine.* NY: Basic Books.

Steinmetz, K., Kushi, L., Bostick, R., Folsum, A., & Potter, J. (1994). Vegetables, fruits, and colon cancer in the Iowa Women's Health Study. *American Journal of Epidemiology, 139,* 1–15.

Stevinson, C., & Ernst, E.(1999). Safety of *Hypericum* in patients with depression: a comparison with conventional antidepressants. *CNS Drugs, 11*(2), 125–132.

Stich, H. (1992). Teas and tea components as inhibitors of carcinogen formation in model systems and man. *Preventive Medicine, 21,* 377–384.

Stickel, F., &Seitz, H.K. The efficacy and safety of comfrey. *Public Health Nutrition, 3*(4A), 501-508.

Stimpel, M., Proksch, A., Wagner, H., & Lohmann-Matthes, M. (1984). Macrophage activation and induction of macrophage cytotoxicity by purified polysaccharide fractions from the plant *Echinacea purpurea. Infection and Immunity, 46*(3), 845–849.

Stoll, W. (1987). Phytotherapy influences atrophic vaginal epithelium. *Therapeutikon, 1,* 23. Cited in S. Lieberman (1998). A review of the effectiveness of *Cimicifuga racemosa* (black cohosh) for the symptoms of menopause. *Journal of Women's Health, 7*(5):525–529.

Stough, C., Clarke, J., Lloyd, J., & Nathan, P. J. (2001). Neuropsychological changes after 30-day *Ginkgo biloba* administration in healthy participants. *International Journal of Neuropsychopharmacology, 4*(2), 131–134.

Sunter, W. (1991). Warfarin and garlic [letter]. *Pharmacological Journal, 246,* 722.

Sur, P., Das, M., Gomes, A., Vedasiromoni, J. R., Sahu, N. P., Banerjee, S., Sharma, R. M., & Ganguly, D. K. (2001). *Trigonella foenum graecum* (fenugreek) seed extract as an antineoplastic agent. *Phytotherapy Research, 15*(3), 257–259.

Taussig, S., & Batkin, S. (1988). Bromelain, the enzyme complex of pineapple and its clinical application. An update. *Journal of Ethnopharmacology, 22,* 191–203.

Teucher, T., Obertreis, B., Ruttkowski, B., & Schmitz, H. (September 1996). Cytokine secretion in whole blood of healthy volunteers after oral ingestion of an *Urtica dioca L.* leaf extract. *Arzneimittelforschung, 46*(9), 906–910. Cited in *HerbalGram, 49*:62.

Tompkins, P., & Bird, C. (1973). *The Secret Life of Plants.* New York: Harper & Row.

Traditional Medicinals Gallup Survey. (1999). Cited in *HerbalGram* (2000), *48,* 66.

Tubaro, A., Tragni, E., DelNegro, P., Galli, C., & Loggia. (1987). Anti-inflammatory activity of a polysaccharidic fraction of echinacea angustifolia. *Journal of Pharmacognosy and Pharmacology, 39,* 567–569.

Tyler, V. (March 1996). Herbs and health care in the twenty-first century. *Herbs for Health,* 10–12.

Tyler, V. (1993). *The honest herbal.* Binghamton, NY: Pharmaceutical Products Press.

Tyler, V. (1994). *Herbs of choice.* Binghamton, NY: Pharmaceutical Products Press.

Tyler, V. (1996). What pharmacists should know about herbal remedies. *Journal of the American Pharmaceutical Association, NS36*(1), 29–37.

Ulrich, L. T. (1991). *A midwife's tale: The life of Martha Ballard, based on her diary,* 1785–1812. New York: Alfred A. Knopf.

United States Food and Drug Administration Center for Food Safety and Applied Nutrition. (December 1, 1995). Dietary Supplement Health and Education Act of 1994. [on-line], Available: Hostname: vm.cfsan.fda.gov/-dms/dietsupp.html.

Upton, R. (1999). International Symposium of the European Scientific Cooperative on Phytotherapy (ESCOP), London, October 1998. *HerbalGram, 46,* 60.

Upton, R. (Ed.) (1999). Valerian (*Valerian officinalis*). *American herbal* CA: Soquel.

Velasquez, M. T., & Bhathena, S. J. (2001). Dietary phytoestrogens: A possible role in renal disease protection. *American Journal of Kidney Diseases, 37*(5), 1056–1068.

Verbuta, A., & Cojocaru, I. (1996). Research to achieve a homeopathic lotion. *Revista Medico-Chirurgicala a Societatii de Medici si Naturalisti din Iasi, 100*(1–2), 172–174.

Vereshchagin, I., Geskina, O., & Bukhteeva, E. (1982) Increasing antibiotic therapy efficacy with adaptogens in children suffering from dysentery. *Antibiotiki, 27*(1), 65–69. Cited by F. Brinker. *Herb contraindications and drug interactions,* 2nd edition. (1998) OR: Eclectic Medical Publications.

Vibes, J., Lasserre, B., Gleye, J., & Declume, C. (1994). Inhibition of thromboxane A2 biosynthesis in vitro by the main components of Crataegus oxyacanthan (Hawthorne) flower heads. *Prostaglandins Leukot Essential Fatty Acids* 50:173–175 [Medline].

Vogt, H., et al. (1988). Melissenextrakt bei Herpes simplex. *Der Allgemeinarzt, 13,* 3–15, 1991.

Vogel, V. (1970). *American Indian medicine.* Norman, OK: University of Oklahoma Press.

Volz, H. P., & Kieser, M. (1997). Kava-kava extract WS 1490 versus placebo in anxiety disorders—A randomized placebo-controlled 25-week outpatient trial. *Pharmacopsychiatry, 30,* 1–5.

Wang, Z., Cheng, S., & Zhou, C. Antimutagenic activity of green tea polyphenols. *Mutation Research, 223,* 273–289.

Warshafsky, S., Kamer, R., & Sivak, S. (1993). Effect of garlic on total serum cholesterol. *Annals of Internal Medicine, 119*:599–605.

Wasser, S., & Weis, A. (1999). Therapeutic effects of substances occurring in higher *Basidiomycetes* mushrooms: a modern perspective. *Critical Review of Immunology, 19*(1), 65–96.

Weed, S. (1996). *Breast cancer? Breast health! The wise woman way.* Woodstock, NY: Ash Tree.

Weed, S. (1986). *The childbearing year.* Woodstock, NY: Ash Tree.

Weed, S. (1992). *Menopausal Years: The Wise Woman Way.* Woodstock, NY: Ash Tree.

Weisman, E. (October 1994). New ways to keep people healthy. *Trustee,* 8–12.

Weiss, G., & Weiss, S. (1985). *Growing and using the healing herbs.* Emmaus, PA: Rodale Press.

Weiss, R. F. (1988). *Herbal medicine.* Beaconsfield, England: Beaconsfield Publishers Ltd.

Weizman, Z., Alkrinawi, S., Goldfarb, D., & Bitran, C. (1993). Efficacy of herbal tea preparation in infantile colic. *The Journal of Pediatrics, 122,* 650–652.

Werbach, M., & Murray, M. (1994). *Botanical influences on illness: A source book of clinical research.* CA: Third Line Press.

Wesnes, K A., Ward, T., McGinty, A., & Petrini, O. (2000). The memory enhancing effects of a *Ginkgo biloba/Panax ginseng* combination in healthy middle-aged volunteers. *Psychopharmacology (Berlin), 152*(4), 353–361.

Wichtl, M. (Ed.). (1994). *Herbal drugs and phytopharmaceuticals*. Boca Raton, FL: CRC Press.

Willey, L., Mady, S., Cobaugh, D., & Wax, P. (1995). Valerian overdose: A case report. *Veterinarian and Human Toxicology, 37*(4), 364–365.

Williams, CA, Goldstone, F., & Greenham, J. (1996. Flavonoids, cinnamic acids and coumarins from the different tissues and medicinal preparations of *Taraxacum officinale*. Phytochemistry, *42*(1), 121–127.

Wilt, T. J., et al (1998). Saw palmetto extracts for treatment of benign prostatic hyperplasia. *Journal of the American Medical Association, 158*(18), 1604–1609.

Winship, K. A. (1991). Toxicity of comfrey. *Adverse Drug Reactions Toxicology Review, 10*(1), 47–59.

Wobling, R., & Leonhardt, K. (1994). Local therapy of Herpes simplex with dried extract from *Melissa officinalis*. Phytomedicine, *1*, 25–31.

Wood, R. (1999). *The new whole foods encyclopedia*. New York: Penguin.

World Health Organization. (1999). *WHO monographs on selected medicinal plants*. Vol. 1. Geneva: The Organization.

World Health Organization Programme on Traditional Medicines. 1991. Guideline for the Assessment of Herbal Medicines. Geneva: WHO, reprinted in *HerbalGram* (*1993*), 28, 17–20.

Woywodt, A., Hermann, A., Choi, M., Goebel, U., & Luft, F. (2000). Turkish pepper (extra hot). *Postgraduate Medical Journal, 76*(897), 426–428.

Yarnell, E. (June 1998). Stinging nettle: a modern view of an ancient healing plant. *Alternative and Complementary Therapies*, 180–186.

Yeoh, K., Kang, Y., Yap, I., Guan, R., Tan, C. C., Wee, A., & Teng, C. H. Chili protects against aspirin-induced gastroduodenal mucosal injury in humans. *Digestive Diseases and Sciences, 40*(3), 580–583.

Yoshida, Y., Wang, M., Liu, J., Shan, B., & Yamashita, U. (1997). Immunomodulating activity of Chinese medicinal herbs and *Oldenlandra diffusa* in particular. *International Immunopharmacology, 19*(7), 359–370.

Youngkin, E., & Israel, D. (October 1996). A review and critique of common herbal alternative therapies. *Nurse Practitioner*, 39–45.

Yongchaiyudha, S., Rungpitarangsi, V., Bunyapraphatsara, N., et al. (1996). Antidiabetic activity of *Aloe vera* L. Juice. Clinical trial in new cases of diabetes mellitus. *Phytomedicine, 3*(3), 241–243.

Zafriri, D., Ofek, I., Adar, R., Pocino, M., & Sharon, N. (1989). Inhibitory activity of cranberry juice on adherence of type 1 and type P fimbriated *Escherichia coli* to eucaryotic cells. *Antimicrobial Agents and Chemotherapy, 33*(1), 92–98.

Zhang, J., Fu, S., Liu, S., Mao, T., & Xiu, R. (2000). The therapeutic effect of *Ginkgo biloba* extract in SHR rats and its possible mechanisms based on cerebral microvascular flow and vasomotion. *Clinical Hemorheology and Microcirculation, 23*(2–4), 133–138.

Zhang, W., & Li Wan Po (1994). The effectiveness of topically applied capsaicin. A meta-analysis. *European Journal of Clinical Pharmacology, 46*(6), 517–522.

Zhu, M., Wong, P. Y., & Li, R. C. (1999). Effect of oral administration of fennel (Foeniculum vulgare) on ciprofloxacin absorption and disposition in the rat. *Journal of Pharmacy and Pharmacology, 51*(12), 1391–1396.

Zi, X., & Agarwal, R. (1999). Silibinin decreases prostate-specific antigen with cell growth inhibition via GI arrest, leading to differentiation of prostate carcinoma cells: Implication s for prostate cancer intervention. *Proceedings of the National Academy of Sciences of the United States of America, 96*(13), 7490–7495.

Zi, X., Zhang, J., Agarwal, R., & Pollack, M. (2000). Silibinin up-regulates insulin-like growth factor-binding protein 3 expression and inhibits proliferation of androgen-independent prostate cancer cells. *Cancer Research, 60*(20), 5617–5620.

Zia, T., Hasnain, S. N., & Hasan, S. K. (2001). Evaluation of the oral hypoglycaemic effect of *Trigonella foenum-graecum L.* (methi) in normal mice. *Journal of Ethnopharmacology, 75*, 191195.

RESOURCES

BOOKS AND JOURNALS ON HERBAL MEDICINE

Blumenthal, M., Busse, W, Goldberg, A., Gruenwald, J., Hall, T., Riggins, C., & Rister, R. (Eds.). (1998). *The complete German Commission E monographs: Therapeutic guide to herbal medicines* (S. Klein & R. Rister, Trans). Austin, TX: American Botanical Council; Newton, MA: Integrative Medicine Communications.

Blumenthal, M., Goldberg, A, & Brinckmann, J. (Eds.). (2000). *Herbal medicine expanded Commission E monographs.* Austin, TX: American Botanical Council; Newton, MA: Integrative Medicine Communications.

Bown, D. (1995). *The herb society of America encyclopedia of herbs and their uses.* New York: Dorling Kindersley Publishing.

Bratman, S, & Kroll, D. (2000). *The natural pharmacist: Your complete guide to illnesses and their natural remedies.* Roseville, CA: Prima Publishing.

Brinker, F. (1998). *Herb contraindications and drug interactions.* (2nd ed.). Sandy, OR: Eclectic Medical Publications.

Duke, J. (1985). *Handbook of medicinal herbs.* Boca Raton, FL: CRC Press.

Gladstar, R. (1993). *Herbal healing for women.* New York: Simon & Schuster.

HerbalGram (Peer-reviewed scientific journal on herbal medicines).

Herbs for Health (Journal with feature articles by herb specialists for medicinal, culinary, and gardening purposes).

Hoffman, D. (1994). *The information sourcebook of herbal medicine.* Freedom, CA: The Crossing Press.

Hoffman, D. (1992). *The new holistic herbal.* Rockport, MA.: Element, Inc.

Kowalchik, C., & Hylton, W. (Eds.). (1987). *Rodale's illustrated encyclopedia of herbs.* Emmaus, PA: Rodale Press.

McCaleb, R., Leigh, E., & Morien, K. (2000). *The encyclopedia of popular herbs.* Roseville, CA: Prima Health.

McGuffin, M., Hobbs, C., Upton, R., & Goldberg, A. (1997). *Botanical safety handbook.* Boca Raton, FL: CRC Press.

Murray, M. (1991). *The healing power of herbs.* Roseville, CA: Prima Publishing.

Murray, M. A natural alternative to estrogen for menopause. *Cimicifuga* extract (Black cohosh). Health Counselor [publisher].

Murray, M., & Werbach, M. (1994). *Botanical influences on illness.* Tarzana, CA: Third Line Press.

Ody, P. (1993). *The complete medicinal herbal.* New York: Dorling Kinderlsey Publishing.

Ottariano, S. (1999). *Medicinal herbal therapy: A pharmacist's viewpoint.* North Hampton, NH: Nicolin Fields Publishing.

PDR for herbal medicines (1998). Montvale, NJ: Medical Economics Company.

Prescriber's Letter (2000). *Natural Medicines Comprehensive Database.* Stockton, CA: Therapeutic Research Faculty.

The Review of Natural Products (formerly The Lawrence Review). St. Louis, MO: Facts & Comparisons; updated monthly.

Scott, J. (1990). *Natural medicine for children.* London: Gaia.

Tyler, V. (1994). *Herbs of choice: The therapeutic use of phytomedicinals.* Binghamton, NY: Haworth Press.

Tyler, V. (1993). *The honest herbal.* Binghamton, NY: Haworth Press.

Weed, S. (1986). *The childbearing year.* Woodstock, NY: Ash Tree.

Weed, S. (1992). *Menopausal years: The wise woman way.* Woodstock, NY: Ash Tree.

Weiss, G., & Weiss, S. (1985). *Growing and using the healing herbs.* Emmaus, PA: Rodale Press.

Weiss, R. F. (1988). *Herbal medicine.* Beaconsfield, England: Beaconsfield Publishers Ltd.

Wichtl, M. (ed). (1994). *Herbal drugs and phytopharmaceuticals.* Boca Raton, FL: CRC Press.

Wood R. (1999). *The new whole foods encyclopedia.* New York: Penguin Press.

World Health Organization monographs on selected medicinal plants. (1999). Albany, NY: World Health Organization.

INTERNET SITES DEALING WITH HERBAL MEDICINE

Algy's Home Page—**www.algy.com/herb**
The Alternative Medicine Homepage—**http://www.pitt.edu/-cbw/altm.html**
American Botanical Council—**http://www.herbalgram.org**
American Herb Association—**www.jps.net/ahaherb/**
American Herbal Pharmacopoeia—**www.herbal-ahp.org**
American Herbalists Guild—**www.healthy.net/herbalists**
Association of Natural Medicine Pharmacists—**http://www.anmp.org**
Bibliographic summary of international CAM information—
    http://cpmcnet.columbia.edu/dept/rosenthal/databases/AM_databases.
    html
Duke, J. Phytochemical and Ethnobotanical Database at the
    AgriculturalResearch Services—**http://www.ars-grin.gov/duke/**
FDA (October 1983). Unsafe Herbs. *FDA Consumer.* [on line]. Available:
    Hostname: **http://lep.cl.msu.edu/msueimp/htdoc/modO3/03900066.**
    html
FDA Special Nutritionals Adverse Event Monitoring System—
    http://vm.cfsan.fda.gov/-dms/aems.html
Herb Research Foundation—**http://www.herbs.org**
Medical Herbalism: A Journal for the Clinical Practitioner—
    http://.medherb.com/
Medicinal and Poisonous Plant Databases—
    http://www/rusticroots.com/mct/

HERB ORGANIZATIONS

AMERICAN BOTANICAL COUNCIL
P.O. Box 144345
Austin, Texas 78714-4345
(512) 926-4900
http://www.herbalgram.org

Wonderful catalog of every herb book imaginable. This organization is the co-publisher of the peer-reviewed journal *HerbalGram*.

AMERICAN HERBALISTS GUILD
P.O. Box 70
Roosevelt, UT 84066
(435) 722-8434
www.healthy.net/herbalists

HERB RESEARCH FOUNDATION
1007 Pearl Street, Suite 200
Boulder, CO 80302
(303) 449–2265
http://www.herbs.org

The HRF's primary goal is education. It provides scientific information to consumers, researchers, and health care professionals. The foundation co-publishes *HerbalGram*, a peer-reviewed journal. This journal is highly recommended for any health-care professional who would like the latest international information and studies about herbs. HRF also publishes *Herbs for Health*, a magazine educating the public about herbs and their uses, with herbal studies, healthy recipes, and more.

NORTHEAST HERBALIST ASSOCIATION
P.O. Box 10
Newport, NY 13416

United Plant Savers
P.O. Box 98
East Barre, VT 05649
(802)479-9825

United Plant Savers is an organization dedicated to saving at-risk native medicinal plants, such as goldenseal, eyebright, *Echinacea angustifolia*, blood root, black cohosh, blue cohosh, American ginseng, lady's slipper, pipsissewa, and osha. Always buy ethically wild-crafted or cultivated plants.

HERB EDUCATION PROGRAMS

For a list of education programs, contact the American Herbalists Guild at (435) 722-8434 or

Sage Mountain Herbal Center
P.O. Box 420
East Barre, VT 05649
(802) 479-9825

Degree Programs

Bastyr University
Admissions/Continuing Education
14500 Juanita Drive N. E.
Bothell, Washington 98011
(425) 602-3070
Naturopathic Doctor (ND) and other degrees

Southwest College of Naturopathic Medicine and Health Sciences
2140 East Broadway Road
Tempe, Arizona 85282
(602) 858-9100
ND, MA in acupuncture

Index